Foods That Fit a Unique You

W. Lee Cowden, MD, MD(H)

Connie Strasheim

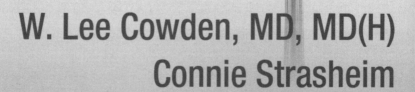

ACIM Press

Foods That Fit a Unique You

Books may be purchased in bulk by contacting
ACIMConnect.com, or Connie Strasheim at: Connie@ConnieStrasheim.com.

Cover Design: Nick Zelinger, NZ Graphics
Interior Design: Rebecca Finkel, F + P Graphic Design
Publisher: ACIM Press
Editor: John Maling, Editing By John
Publishing Consultant: Judith Briles, The Book Shepherd

First edition
Library of Congress Catalog Number: on file
ISBN paperback: 978-0-9961004-2-7
eISBN: 978-0-9961004-3-4

10 9 8 7 6 5 4 3 2 1

First Edition printed in USA, September, 2014

1. Health 2. Nutrition 3. Genetically Altered Organisms (GAOs) 4. Organic Foods

Printed in the USA

Contents

PART TWO
Individualization 61

Foreword

When my friend Connie Strasheim asked me if I would be
willing to write the foreword to her newest book, *Foods That Fit
a Unique You*, co-authored with Dr. W. Lee Cowden, I agreed at
once. First, I was honored to have been included in Ms. Strasheim's
book *Defeat Cancer*, which eloquently presented a variety of
approaches to malignant disease too often ignored by the
mainstream academic medical world. Second, though I do not
personally know Dr. Cowden, I have long been an admirer of his
pioneering work in nutritional medicine and stress reduction.

Happily, through this effort, these authors together have
produced a wonderfully insightful book that, though brief in
length, provides an enormous amount of on-target, useful, and
practical information important for anyone with an interest in
nutrition—lay person or healthcare practitioner alike—seeking
to make sense out of the many conflicting dogmas currently
circulating in the world of dietetics and nutritional therapy.
For this effort, carefully and logically constructed, they are to

be commended. Frankly, I was amazed at the wealth of important information they include and how much territory they successfully surveyed in this work.

Ms. Strasheim and Dr. Cowden divide the book into three main sections, beginning with an overview of the problems with our current food supply as we move further into the 21st century.

Here, the authors describe the terrible and worsening problems with depleted soils; the loss of nutrients due to the industrialized processing of foodstuffs, and the increasing reliance on toxic chemicals at every step in food production— from our use of pesticides on crops, to the application of growth stimulants such as estrogen and growth hormones that are given to feedlot cattle, to the processing of foods and their ultimate packaging in toxin-leaching containers.

Then, after this overview, they undertake a much-needed discussion of GMOs; those increasingly pervasive genetically-modified crops, which are now even used on livestock and fish, and created by our agricultural scientists with the hope of "modernizing" and "improving" our food supply. Yet, as is so often the case when foolish man tinkers with nature, they have left us a world of Frankenstein foods that are responsible for a host of documented health problems, from allergies to (it appears) tumors in animals.

The authors present a passionate and scientifically valid argument against such foods; arguments that should fortify those of us that already resist the spread of GMOs, while at the same time, help convince the doubters and skeptics who still hold onto the promise of "Science" over Nature.

Subsequently, Ms. Strasheim and Dr. Cowden embark on a lengthy discussion of the chemistry and biochemistry of different foods, even their effect on metabolism and acid-base balance, and importantly, their influence on brain function. In this section they convincingly introduce the concept of biochemical individuality and "metabolic typing," which is so important to my own practice today.

Put simply, the authors argue that one man's food can indeed be another man's poison, depending on our genetic and physiological makeup, and each of us requires a diet and nutritional program designed with our particular biological needs in mind for optimal health. I agreed wholeheartedly with this concept, best summed up as "one size does not fit all" and that a diet suitable for one person may send another into catastrophic poor health. For acknowledging these principles, and for presenting their arguments so thoughtfully, they indeed deserve credit.

Too often, experts in the world of nutrition and dietetics, both conventional and alternative, routinely proclaim to the world with dictatorial certainty the newest perfect diet—be it low carb, high carb, low fat or no fat—which all of us, whatever our size, shape, genetics or the geographic origins of our ancestors, should follow. Such pronouncements routinely sell millions of books, but most often leave the reader befuddled and confused because the latest tome contradicts the tenets of the previous best-selling, "perfect" diet book. Ms. Strasheim and Dr. Cowden help put the confusion to rest with their suggestion that our own dietary needs may vary enormously from those of our neighbor just down the street.

I am particularly pleased to find a section devoted to my late mentor, the eccentric but most brilliant William Donald Kelley, DDS, the Texas-based dentist, who, during the 1960s and 1970s, developed a comprehensive nutritional program for the treatment of cancer and other serious degenerative diseases. Although poor Dr. Kelley was harassed for years by various regulatory authorities, he did successfully treat some of the most aggressive cancers, including pancreatic cancer, as my lengthy five-year investigation of his practice and patients documented. Sadly, he went to his grave never achieving his dream that his work might receive at least a modicum of academic recognition.

I am also happy that this book provides a discussion of the psychological and spiritual aspects of healing. Too often, those of us in the alternative world are guilty of the same sins as our conventional medical practitioner colleagues, seeing humans more as lab rats for which the magic vitamin or food will make the ultimate difference in health. Though surely, as a practitioner of nutritional medicine myself, we in the field appreciate the importance of right diet and properly designed supplement programs. Yet, as the authors point out, for optimal health we need to consider the psychological issues, especially the psychological stressors, that inevitably contribute to disease.

Shortly after I met Dr. Kelley in 1981, I naively asked him what percentage of disease he considered to be purely nutritional, what percentage psychological and what percentage spiritual. He answered wisely from his long experience with patients, "That's simple; it's 100 percent nutritional" (which was the answer I expected). Then after a pause, he continued, "It's also 100 percent psychological, and 100 percent spiritual, in every patient I have treated, and in every patient you will treat." Ms. Strasheim and Dr. Cowden understand that precept fully, arguing in their book that psychological conflicts need to be addressed, while including simple methods for dealing with difficult stressful situations.

This is a gem of a book for many reasons, and one that will hopefully receive wide readership. The authors manage, within the confines of a relatively short book, to provide the essentials of nutritional biochemistry, help unravel the confusion rampant in the alternative world of diet and nutrition, bring in concepts of stress-reduction, and provide simple tips for food preparation that can be adopted to any home or kitchen. They cover the nutritional and healing bases well—convincingly and wisely.

—Nicholas J. Gonzalez, MD

Nicholas J. Gonzalez, MD is author of *One Man Alone: An Investigation of Nutrition, Cancer, and William Donald Kelley* and *What Went Wrong: The Truth Behind the Clinical Trial of the Enzyme Treatment of Cancer,* among others.

Part One

Principles of a Healthy Diet

Forty-two-year-old Sarah frequently visited her primary care dotor for a prescription to relieve her random but ongoing symptoms—which included depression, brain fog, fatigue, upper back pain, constipation, irritable bowel, and acid reflux. She didn't feel sick, really—just not energetic or at her best most days.

Today, she found herself once again in the waiting room of Dr. Pharma, her primary physician. She felt drowsy, irritable and downcast. Wasn't the antidepressant that Dr. Pharma had given her supposed to alleviate some of these symptoms? So why didn't it seem to be doing much?

If he could just help me to lose weight, she reasoned, I'm sure my mood and energy would be much better. So here she was again, hoping that he might be able to give her yet another prescription—this time, for weight loss. She despised the thought of having to add yet another medication to her already broad assortment of drugs—amitryptilene, acetaminophen, ibupofren, and a variety of antacids—but she had been packing on the pounds rapidly in recent years, and she feared becoming obese if she didn't do something about it.

Surely Dr. Pharma could do something for her. Anyway, it wasn't like she was eating Twinkies for breakfast every day—she had faithfully tried a multitude of diets; South Beach, Atkin's, Weight Watcher's, and others—but none had worked long-term.

She had eliminated sweets and desserts from her diet— even bread, opting instead for canned vegetable soups, low-fat, low-calorie microwaveable dinners, and artificially sweetened yogurt, non-fat milk and diet bars. She faithfully ate vegetables and fruits at least twice daily, especially carrots and beets, since she had read somewhere that they were high in antioxidants. She tried to stay away from red meat, since Dr. Pharma had told her that red meat would increase her already high levels of unhealthy cholesterol.

But consuming low-calorie, or low carbohydrate food, or simply food in small amounts, did nothing for her. Yes, she felt like she really needed a drug now. Surely Dr. Pharma could help her. Or at least she hoped ….

If Sarah sounds like you, or somebody that you know, you are not alone! Many people today suffer from undiagnosed aches and pains, fatigue, and other symptoms, and are pudgy or over-weight. Maybe you are like Sarah, and you strive to be well, but it feels like no matter what you or your doctors do, you either feel terrible or less than your best, and you can't seem to lose weight.

Sarah's scenario has become extraordinarily common among people of all ages today, and unbeknownst to many of us, our diets are (still) a big reason why many of us are overweight, sluggish, sick and tired. You might say, "But I don't eat that much!" or "I eat pretty well."

If you are like many Americans, you probably think that you are eating at least some of the right foods, but you are really sabotaging your efforts because you either don't know, or pay attention to, what's really in your so-called "healthy" foods. Or you may be eating certain foods just because the media or your doctor said that they are good for you, when in reality they are the reason for your grouchiness, sleeplessness, fatigue, brain fog and the excess inches on your waist.

You don't have to be like Sarah, going from doctor to doctor and taking prescriptions, or doing the latest fad diet, in the hopes that they will make you thinner, happier, and more functional. Anyway, drugs only make most problems worse, and never get to their root cause.

In this book, you'll learn how to make healthy food choices and find the foods that best fit you, as a unique person with unique dietary needs. As you follow these guidelines, we believe that your symptoms and weight problems will diminish or disappear, and you'll find yourself experiencing better health than you ever have before.

Why? Because food is medicine to the body, and when you eat the foods that are right for your specific needs and body type, you will tend to be well. Many diseases are caused, at least in part, by eating the wrong foods but we don't usually attribute our symptoms to what we put into our mouths everyday. In the following pages, you will see how and why eating the right foods can literally transform your life. So read on!

CHAPTER ONE

Discover the Foods That Are Right for You

Hippocrates said, "Let your food be your medicine, and let your medicine be your food."

Food should be medicine to the body, but our food supply isn't what it used to be. Eating well in today's toxic, fast-paced world has become a challenge, and our hectic lifestyles preclude us from being able to spend more than a few minutes in the kitchen to prepare healthy meals. And as our waistlines expand and we become increasingly sluggish we become lost in a sea of one-size-fits-all diet books, confused by a multitude of dietary guidelines that all promise to make us fit, energetic and healthy.

No wonder some of us feel as though we need a PhD to know how to eat well. Sadly, despite the rows of dietary books that line some of our bookshelves, few of us really feel great, partly because we are (still) eating the wrong stuff.

Our bodies and minds require proper nutrition to function well, and eating the right food is essential for wellness. Despite the chemically toxic world that we live in, we believe that it's possible to find foods that promote health, vitality and a trim waistline, but we must know how to identify them.

Individually, each of us is unique, and for that reason the foods that each of us need for health, happiness and a slender body can't be found in one-size-fits-all diet books.

In our journey towards wellness, and as we mention in the first book of this series, *Create a Toxin-Free Body & Home Starting Today,* we believe that it is possible to move past survival mode, and thrive—in body, mind and spirit—if we are simply given the proper tools. One of those tools is the right diet for our unique body type—our unique biochemistry.

Wellness doesn't have to mean an absence of symptoms or mere functionality. If you give your body the right foods, you can experience strength, vitality and well-being on a daily basis. You can even attain your ideal weight without having to count calories.

Food isn't just medicine for the body, but also the soul and spirit, since eating the right cuisine enables all aspects of our being to function more fully in harmony with one another— because it isn't just the body that requires nutrition, but the mind, emotions and spirit, as well.

Individually, each of us is unique, and for that reason the foods that each of us need for health, happiness and a slender body can't be found in one-size-fits-all diet books. Yet finding foods that fit your unique biochemistry doesn't require a PhD degree. It is not that complex!

Studies are useful, but we are not a study and we don't all respond to the same dietary protocols that have had successful outcomes for some. No "study" has ever provided 100 percent success, even among the test subjects. Results are always couched in statistical terms.

It requires that you know a little about who you are and how you feel after eating different foods, and that you understand some general guidelines about how and what to eat. It also requires knowing how to identify healthy foods in the grocery store, and how to prepare them, which doesn't have to be a chore if you take the time to read the basic guidelines outlined in *Foods That Fit a Unique You.*

The benefits of the journey to wellness, such as joy, energy and the ability to be the kind of person that you want to be, and do the things that you want to do in life—are attainable if you are just given the proper tools. We all need wisdom to navigate the toxic world in which we live and to seek out what's beneficial for us, amidst the abundance—literally, a Noah's flood—of information that's out there on the Internet, in diet books, on TV and elsewhere.

It's essential that we eat clean, nutrient-dense, unadulterated, unprocessed food to be well. In this book, we teach you how to identify that kind of food. It is just as essential, however, that we teach you how to discover the foods that are right for you, as the unique person that you are with your own special set of needs. These needs may contradict medical studies, other diet books, and even your doctor's recommendations! (By the way, few doctors are taught much about diet or nutrition in medical school.)

Just because one type of diet worked for one person, doesn't mean it will work for you. Forget the books that promise that if you just eat your peas and carrots, you will be well and lose weight—maybe … but maybe not.

The strategies and tools that we offer here are effective because they take into account your health condition, metabolic type, pH and food allergies, among other factors, and are based on Dr. Cowden's experience with thousands of patients.

We don't recommend foods just because studies have shown them to be healthy and nutritious. Studies are useful, but we are not a study and we don't all respond to the same dietary protocols that have had successful outcomes for some. We are complex, and our bodies' needs sometimes defy studies, medicine and logic. Usually, it is our bodies that best dictate what we need.

Studies, diet books, nutritionists, dietitians, integrative medical doctors and other health professionals can all help us seek out the foods that are most beneficial for us. We have relied upon such resources when compiling the information for this book, but our recommendations aren't based on a single set of guidelines or the latest food fad. They are based on

Dr. Cowden's experience with thousands of patients, as well as our own research and personal experience.

> As Hippocrates so wisely preached, food should be medicine for the body. No vitamin supplement can heal the body like food. Food is the fuel on which the body operates, regenerates and repairs itself.

Here we teach you how to identify the foods that will enable you to feel and look your best, based on your individual body type and needs. In Part One, we provide general principles for establishing a clean, healthy diet. In Part Two, we focus on diet individualization, and in Part Three, we offer simple tips for optimal food selection, preparation and digestion.

We hope that *Foods That Fit a Unique You* will help you to discover the healing and life-promoting properties of nutritious food, and that as you follow our suggestions, you will experience a greater level of well-being than you ever have before.

CHAPTER TWO

What's Wrong with Food Today

Once upon a time in history, food healed us, sustained us, and gave us life. But today, food has become a mixed blessing, and only some foods nourish the body, while others contaminate it. Much of our food supply has been polluted by a plethora of toxins, including pesticides, hormones, antibiotics, plastics, and other carcinogens that damage the body and make it susceptible to disease.

Foods in the US contain fewer nutrients than they did just fifty years ago, and most have been genetically modified, manipulated, and biochemically altered into substances that hardly resemble food.

Food should be medicine for the body. No vitamin supplement can heal the body like food. Food is the fuel on which the body operates, regenerates and repairs itself. No supplement can take the place of food, and no manipulating of food can make it better than how God, or nature, created it. To think that we can mess with God's, or if you prefer, nature's, original design for food by altering its DNA and adding toxins to it that the body wasn't designed to process, and not pay a price for it, is naïve.

We are meant to eat food the way it was created in nature, and in the form in which the body was designed to process it. Non-organic food has elements of nutrition to it, but it also harms the body in some way.

Because of these factors, many of us, whether or not we have obvious symptoms of a serious illness, have multiple nutrient deficiencies and are overweight and overloaded with environmental toxins that are affecting our body's biochemical processes. We may not be sick (yet), but the healthy integrity of our bodies may be starting to quietly unravel, unbeknownst to us, and this unraveling is manifesting itself in nagging health problems that we suffer from, such as back pain, recurring headaches, chronic constipation or low energy—symptoms that most of us attribute to stress and the aches and pains of daily living, but which are really the result of eating the wrong foods.

Still others of us may be struggling to overcome a major chronic illness, thinking that it's purely an infection or a problem of genetic weakness that's making us ill; something we can blame on our parents or grandparents, when in truth, our diets are a principal source of the problem. Or maybe we are battling weight gain, believing it to be the natural result of aging.

Regardless, it's difficult to feel your best, maintain an ideal weight, or recover from symptoms when you aren't consuming clean, healthy foods that are right for your body.

In today's toxic world, and no matter your current health status or body type, it's essential to eat organic food. Eating organic used to be seen as a luxury, or even a fad—for people who wanted to stay super healthy. Yet the truth is that the only real food anymore is organic. All other food contains harmful amounts of pesticides, herbicides, antibiotics and hormones, among other manmade chemicals that our bodies have not been designed to process. We're not supposed to eat chemicals and drugs on a daily basis. We'll get fat, sick and tired if we do. It's that simple.

We are meant to eat food the way it was created in nature, and in the form in which the body was designed to process it. Non-organic food has elements of nutrition to it, but it also harms the body in some way. Eating organic food may be expensive, but so is being sick or overweight. It's harder to dig yourself out of the hole of illness than spend a few extra dollars to just stay out of it. Trust us, we've been there!

Genetically modified organisms (GMOs) have been linked to a multitude of health conditions and can either be a contributing or main factor to disease.

Fifty years ago, most of us might have been able to get away with consuming food that wasn't labeled "organic," because the food supply was very different back then—cleaner and more nutrient-dense.

For example, studies worldwide have revealed that the nutritional content of our food has fallen substantially in recent decades. Studies published in *Food Magazine* (January–March 2006), the *Journal of the American College of Nutrition* (Vol. 23:6, 2004) and *Life Extension Magazine* (March 2001), revealed that three spears of broccoli in 1999 contained only 48.3 mg of calcium, whereas in 1951 they contained 130 mg. That's two-thirds less calcium in only 48 years! The Vitamin A content of broccoli in 1999 was only 1,542 IU; in 1951 it was 3,500 IU.

Today, those numbers would be even lower. A potato in 1951 contained 17 mg of Vitamin C; in 1999, it was 7.25 mg. It makes you wonder whether there is any Vitamin C left in potatoes today. A linear extrapolation—strictly a guess— suggests that there could be even 30 percent less in 2014 than in 1999. According to these same studies, the nutrient content of other foods has also fallen substantially, as well.

In general, organic food contains higher levels of nutrients than non-organic food, depending on where it came from. Fruits and vegetables that are picked prematurely and shipped across thousands of miles, for example, will not usually be as nutrient-dense as food that is locally grown and picked ripe. But locally grown organic food will tend to be higher in nutrients than locally produced non-organic food.

Fruits and vegetables today are nutrient-deficient partly because of modern industrial farming practices, which deplete the soil of nutrients that should end up in the food that's grown there. Extensive plowing, using chemical pesticides and fertilizers, and failing to rotate crops and replace depleted soils with organic materials, all cause essential nutrients to be removed from the soil. Nutrient-deficient soil means nutrient-deficient food.

Meat and other animal products are also nutrient-deficient because conventionally raised farm animals are fed foods that they aren't designed to eat. For instance, cows are given corn and even the byproducts of other cows. They are also forced to live in unnatural, confining and toxic environments. This degrades the quality of their meat. Later in *Foods That Fit a Unique You,* we describe other problems with conventionally raised livestock.

For this reason, it's best to consume healthy, organic foods, preferably those which come from small, local farms that rely on traditional organic farming practices such as free-ranging of animals, crop rotation, composting, green manure and biological, rather than chemical, pest control. Organic farming methods sustain the health of the soil, ecosystem and people.

In the chapters in Part One, we describe in greater detail some of the dangers of eating non-organic food, and then share some simple guidelines for how to choose healthy, organic food. These guidelines should form the basis of any healthy food plan. After that, in Part Two, we'll teach you how to choose foods that will meet your body's unique biochemical needs.

CHAPTER THREE

Foods that Make Everyone Sick, Fat and Tired

GENETICALLY MODIFIED (GM) FOOD

Almost all corn, wheat and soy in the United States is now genetically modified, and the number of foods that are becoming genetically modified is on the rise. Much of the food that's sold in conventional (non-organic) supermarkets is also genetically modified.

Genetically modified organisms (GMOs) have been linked to a multitude of health conditions and can either be a contributing or main factor in disease. Such is the concern among scientists about the dangers of GMOs that more than 800 scientists from eighty-four countries have signed the Open Letter from World Scientists to All Governments Concerning Genetically Modified Organisms. This letter, which was submitted to the UN, the World Trade Organization, and the U.S. Congress, emphasizes the serious hazards of GMOs.

Additionally, many U.S. Food and Drug Administration (FDA) scientists have communicated deep concern about the dangerous effects of GMOs upon health, but their voices have been muted by the agricultural biotechnology industry (companies like Monsanto) which has, through its lobbying efforts, convinced the public and the FDA that GMOs aren't bad for you.

The DNA of GMO food is foreign to the body, which means that the body cannot effectively digest it.

Unfortunately, people with financial ties to the biotechnology companies that are responsible for creating GMOs also work in positions of authority at the FDA and U.S. Department of Agriculture (USDA) which creates a conflict of interest between the biotech firms and those agencies. The FDA and USDA are supposed to protect consumer health, but they can't effectively do this when those in authority within these organizations have a financial stake in the success of agricultural biotechnology companies, and therefore, GMOs. Biotechnology representatives influence the laws regarding our food supply, and their interests directly conflict with consumer health.

GMOs have been proven to damage the body in multiple ways. First, they can cause allergic reactions, some of which are life-threatening. In 1989, GMO L-tryptophan caused severe allergic reactions in thousands of people, and was removed from the market after dozens of people died from it.

In a 1999 study, researchers at York Nutritional Laboratory in Great Britain discovered that reactions to soy had increased by 50 percent from the previous year, and that these reactions were most likely caused by genetically modified soy, which had been recently exported from the United States into Great Britain. Many people in the US are also allergic to soy, and not because soy in general is bad for you, but because it is genetically-modified.

GMOs also cause or increase the severity of autoimmune disease. The DNA of GMO food is foreign to the body, which means that the body cannot effectively digest it. Instead, the food passes through the intestinal wall into the bloodstream, where it causes inflammation and triggers autoimmune responses. Inflammation sets the stage for a variety of disease processes to occur, including cancer, and is the underlying precursor for most illnesses.

When we consume excessive amounts of corn, our susceptibility to autoimmune conditions and food allergies increases.

More recent studies have continued to reveal the damaging effects of GMO food. For instance, a 2012 study, "Long term toxicity of a Roundup herbicide and a Roundup-tolerant genetically modified maize," the results of which were published in the medical journal *Food and Chemical Toxicology*, revealed GMO corn and the herbicide Roundup to cause severe health problems in mice. GMO corn and the herbicide Roundup are produced by the biotechnology giant Monsanto and used on crops throughout the US.

Mice are used in scientific studies because they are genetically similar to humans, and what happens in mice tests often indicates what would also happen if the same substance were tested on humans.

In this study, mice exposed to Roundup-resistant GMO corn developed tumors, severe kidney problems and liver congestion. In addition, this so-called food altered the animals' hormonal balance and disabled their pituitary glands, which is the master gland for hormonal regulation in the body.

Whenever we reference studies, we first look at whether the study was financed by an entity with a financial interest or tie to GMO technology. Study results may not be valid unless the studies are conducted by disinterested scientists, since studies can sometimes be created to favor a biased outcome.

If you don't trust studies, we encourage you to talk to a holistic or integrative medical doctor for a firsthand report about how GMOs damage the body, since these doctors often witness healing in their patients whenever their patients switch from GMO to organic food. Many doctors, including Dr. Cowden, have regularly seen their patients recover more quickly from illness when they remove GMO food from their diets.

Consumer polls have shown that most people wouldn't buy food if they knew that it was genetically modified. Recently, bills were proposed in California and Washington that would have required food manufacturers to label GMO food, but the bills failed because the companies that produce GMO food spent millions of dollars in advertising to lobby consumers and make the proponents of GMO labeling look bad.

GMO CORN

Nearly all corn and soy produced in the US is heavily subsidized by the government, in addition to being genetically modified, which means that these foods are found in a multitude of other food products because they are cheap. A large percentage of the foods sold in most conventional grocery stores contain ingredients made from corn. When we consume excessive amounts of corn, our susceptibility to autoimmune conditions and food allergies increases.

Corn and corn by-products are found in many boxed and canned foods, but also in the diets of livestock, poultry and farm-raised fish, because they are inexpensive. This is a problem because cows and fish weren't designed to eat corn! It's like giving human beings dog food and expecting them to feel and function well on it. Corn makes cows sick, and the quality of their meat becomes heavily adulterated as a result of it.

Non-GMO soy can be healthy for some people, when eaten in moderation and consumed in healthy fermented foods such as miso, natto and tempeh.

Studies show that when cows are fed a corn-based diet, they develop enlarged livers and infections, which must then be treated with antibiotics. When we consume their meat, we also end up ingesting whatever they were fed—including those antibiotics.

Michael Pollen, a famous journalist and the bestselling author of *The Omnivore's Dilemma*, traveled to farms all around the US to learn about how food is grown, produced and distributed in America. In a March 2002 *New York Times* article entitled "Power Steer," he shares what he learned about cows that are given corn:

> A corn diet can also give a cow acidosis. Unlike that in our own highly acidic stomachs, the normal pH of a rumen (cow stomach) is neutral. Corn makes it unnaturally acidic, however, causing a kind of bovine heartburn, which in some cases can kill the animal but usually just makes it sick. Acidotic animals go off their feed, pant and salivate excessively, paw at their bellies and eat dirt. The condition can lead to diarrhea, ulcers, bloat, liver disease and a general weakening of the immune system that leaves the animal vulnerable to everything from pneumonia to feedlot polio.
>
> Corn also causes cows' meat to become disproportionately high in omega-6 fatty acids. Omega-6 fatty acids aren't harmful when we consume them in moderation, but most of us have an excess of omega-6 fatty acids in our bodies. These fats cause inflammation and obesity, and are linked to a multitude of degenerative diseases, including cancer, autoimmune illness, and irritable bowel and metabolic syndromes.

Meat from animals that are fed corn and other grains is estimated to contain only 15 to 50 percent of the amount of inflammation-lowering and health-promoting omega-3 fatty acids that are found in meat from grass-fed livestock. The meat of grass-fed animals also has higher levels of Vitamin E and conjugated linoleic acid, both of which lower cancer risk.

Conventionally raised cows are also fed genetically modified cottonseed, which is heavily sprayed with pesticides and herbicides. These toxic chemicals end up in the animals' feed, then their bodies, and then, you guessed it—your body! Later in *Foods That Fit a Unique You* we describe the harmful effects that pesticides and herbicides have upon the body and how they can compromise our health.

These are just a few reasons why we should all avoid eating corn and conventionally processed meat, poultry and fish.

GMO SOY

Genetically modified soy is another food that most of us would do better without. While non-GMO soy can be healthy and is an important staple of some diets, in the US, almost all soy is genetically modified and is found in a high percentage of processed food products, which means that most of us get way too much of it.

GMO soy also depresses thyroid function and contains plant estrogens that mimic the effects of human estrogen upon the body. Most people in our society have too much estrogen, due to the pseudo-estrogenic effects that environmental toxins have upon the body, so consuming foods that increase estrogen or estrogen-like activity in the body isn't usually a good idea.

In fact, studies have shown that men who consume lots of GMO soy have lowered testosterone levels and decreased sperm counts. When eaten in moderation, however, and consumed in healthy fermented foods such as miso, natto and tempeh, non-GMO soy can be healthy for some people.

Antibiotic and Growth-Hormone-Laden Food

Today, all conventionally raised cows, chickens and even fish are given growth hormones to make them mature faster. Soon these animals, especially salmon, may also be genetically modified.

Besides the question of whether it is ethical to force an animal to mature at twice its natural rate, the growth hormones that these animals are given and which cause them to reach maturity faster end up in the human body and cause numerous health problems such as cancer.

Non-organic meat contains five times as many pesticides as non-organic vegetables, and butter has twenty times the amount of pesticides as non-organic veggies.

Since 1993, all non-organic milk products in the US have contained high levels of Insulin-like Growth Factor-1 (IGF-1), which is a hormone-like substance that stimulates cancer cell growth. High levels of IGF-1 result when cows are given a genetically engineered growth hormone (rBGH) to increase their milk production. Correspondingly, studies published in the *Journal of the National Cancer Institute* and *The Lancet* have since found that people with breast and prostate cancer have higher levels of IGF-1 in their bloodstream. The growth of these cancers is stimulated by artificial hormones such as IGF-1, and evidence suggests that IGF-1 can also stimulate the development of other types of cancer, as well. So drinking non-organic milk or consuming other non-organic milk products is a bad idea!

Just because a food tastes and looks good, doesn't mean that it's healthy. Pharmaceutical and biotech company–sponsored lobbyists have tried to convince people that giving cows and chickens hormones is perfectly safe and that GMOs cause no harm, but scores of scientific studies and many doctors' experiences with their patients indicate otherwise.

Also, as we previously mentioned, the poor cows (and chickens) get sick as a result of their bad diets and are given antibiotics to combat those infections. These antibiotics end up in our bodies when we eat the animal's meat, and kill off vital immune-supportive, friendly bacteria in our guts. These friendly bacteria comprise one of the body's principal defenses against infectious organisms such as bacteria, viruses, yeasts and parasites, which enter the gut through the food, water and air!

Furthermore, conventionally raised livestock have higher levels of stress hormones in their bodies, due to the poor quality of their diets and overcrowded living conditions. So when you eat their meat, you also end up getting these stress hormones in your blood, which then causes an imbalance in your own hormones!

Hormones are important chemical messengers that send signals from glands to tissues and organs, telling them what to do. Any imbalance in the hormones can upset the function of all systems and organs throughout the body, and over time cause illness and weight problems, so ingesting extra hormones is not a good idea!

FOODS THAT CONTAIN PESTICIDES AND HERBICIDES

Pesticides and herbicides, in addition to being found in the feed of conventionally raised livestock, are sprayed on conventionally grown produce, and are another source of disease-promoting inflammation that leads to illness and weight problems.

Among their many detrimental effects upon the body, pesticides create microscopic perforations in the gut and cause leaky gut syndrome, a condition in which undigested whole food particles, instead of being digested by the body, pass through the intestinal lining into the bloodstream where they cause inflammation and allergic reactions.

In my experience, when patients detoxify their bodies of pesticides, they heal more quickly. I teach other clinicians how to do a technique called laser energetic detoxification (LED), which removes pesticides from the body. I have seen patients stop suffering from a multitude of health conditions when they do LED; they heal from insomnia, nervous system problems and other conditions. Pesticides cause de-regulation of the autonomic nervous system (ANS), which then leads to insufficient blood supply to the tissues, malfunction of the hormones and neurotransmitters, poor digestion, and symptoms such as insomnia and chronic fatigue syndrome.

—Dr. Lee Cowden

Pesticides are also associated with some cancers, such as soft-tissue sarcomas, non-Hodgkin's lymphoma, leukemia and prostate, lung and breast cancers. Many studies substantiate these findings. We encourage you to research for yourself on databases such as *PubMed.com* and *GreenMedInfo.com,* the studies that illustrate the harmful effects of pesticides upon the human body.

Contrary to popular belief, most cholesterol doesn't cause heart disease or hardening of the arteries and is actually healthy! It is a vital building block for all cell membranes and is the substance from which Vitamin D and many hormones in the body are made.

Pesticides may damage the body in other ways that scientists are not aware of yet. For instance, one pesticide called Bt (*Bacillus thuringiensis*), which is engineered into GMO foods by biotech companies, is thousands of times more concentrated than natural bug spray, but scientists have yet to test its effects upon the human body!

Finally:

- Non-organic meat contains five times as many pesticides as non-organic vegetables.

- Butter has twenty times the amount of pesticides as non-organic veggies.

- Most non-organic fruits contain more pesticides than vegetables, but less than most non-organic meats and dairy.

If you only have money for some types of organic food, spend it first on animal protein, then secondarily, on fruits, and lastly, vegetables.

Processed Foods that Contain Artificial Additives and Preservatives

Artificial additives and preservatives are another no-no for all of us. They are added to all boxed and canned food products, snacks and fast foods, and are toxic to the body. These substances are added to preserve the shelf life of food, but they won't preserve your life, and may even subtract years from it! An additive isn't good for you if it's a manmade chemical, and chances are, if you can't pronounce the name of an ingredient on a food label, then that ingredient is probably toxic to your body.

Some additives, such as monosodium glutamate (MSG), are so toxic that their fame has spread far and wide (even among those who don't read diet and nutrition books), so food manufacturers are now learning to cleverly re-label them on products so that you won't know what they are.

For instance, MSG, which is linked to neurological disorders, now shows up on ingredient labels as "textured protein," "soy protein isolate" and "natural flavoring"—among other names. It's as if food manufacturers know that most people will associate words like "natural flavoring" and "protein" with healthful substances.

Yet, MSG and many other food additives and preservatives, such as sodium nitrate, BHA, BHT, potassium bromate, aspartame, food colorings, acesulfame-K, carrageenan, and others, are anything but natural to the body, and anything that isn't natural to the body can cause disease-promoting inflammation and lead to DNA damage, hormonal malfunction, obesity, and a variety of chronic, degenerative diseases such as cancer.

Cow Dairy Products

Most cow milk products are contaminated by hormones, antibiotics, and pesticides, and tend to clog the lymphatic vessels of the body. The lymphatic system, with its vessels that run throughout the body, is like a super highway responsible for carrying lymph fluid and toxins and shuttling them out of the body. Milk causes a backup of these toxins, so they can't effectively leave the body and instead get jammed up in the lymphatic system.

Milk can also cause excess mucus in the sinuses, lungs and intestines. It lowers most people's pH (pH will be described later in Chapter Seven, *Food Combining Techniques for Optimal Digestion*), which then makes us prone to contracting infections.

Drinking milk isn't really natural anyway. Humans are the only species of animal that drink milk or the milk of another species after weaning.

Most US dairy products also contain oxycholesterol, which is a type of harmful cholesterol that is often produced by the man-made modification of some foods such as homogenized milk. When you expose the healthy cholesterol in milk to heat and oxygen at the same time, it results in oxycholesterol. Oxycholesterol causes inflammation inside the blood vessels, which results in a hardening of the arteries and increases the risk of heart attacks, strokes, kidney disease and other conditions associated with poor arterial blood flow.

Organic raw milk is okay for some people to drink since it hasn't been homogenized, and doesn't contain harmful chemicals or growth hormones.

Contrary to popular belief, most cholesterol doesn't cause heart disease or hardening of the arteries and is actually healthy. It is a vital building block for all cell membranes and is the substance from which Vitamin D and many hormones in the body are made. Bile salts, which the body uses for digesting and absorbing oils, fats, and fat-soluble vitamins from the intestine, are also made from cholesterol. Oxycholesterol, however, is a different story.

Many years ago, I had a male patient who had a stenosis (abnormal narrowing) of a carotid artery. This artery carries blood to the brain, and this man's artery was more than 80 percent blocked. His cholesterol level was 400 mg/dl, which is very high; twice the normal level.

I don't usually recommend cholesterol drugs to people, but I did for this man because his cholesterol was so high.

He didn't want to take drugs, however, so I put him on a diet that was high in fat-soluble antioxidants, especially tocotrienols (a type of Vitamin E), ascorbyl palmitate (fat-soluble Vitamin C); lipoic acid and some bioflavonoids. These four supplements helped to reduce the oxycholesterol in his blood.

I also put him on a clean, predominantly vegetarian, oxycholesterol-free diet, and had him take protein-digesting enzymes with water 30 minutes before meals, three times daily. Those enzymes digest fibrin and blood clots in the blood vessels.

When I saw this man three months later, his carotid plaque levels had gone down from 80 percent to 20 percent. His total cholesterol level only went down to around 350, however, which proves that cholesterol has very little effect on arterial plaque formation, unless it's in the form of oxycholesterol.

Since seeing this patient, I've treated many other people for high cholesterol, but only by focusing on preventing oxycholesterol production, breaking down arterial fibrin and arterial blood clots. As a result, they have all done well.

— Dr. Lee Cowden

Organic raw milk is okay for some people to drink since it hasn't been homogenized, and doesn't contain harmful chemicals or growth hormones.

FISH CONTAMINATED WITH HEAVY METALS AND OTHER TOXINS

As the world's oceans and lakes become increasingly polluted by radioactive elements and heavy metals such as mercury and other chemical contaminants, sadly, more and more types of fish are becoming unsafe to eat. The mercury in fish, especially, is responsible for contributing to the epidemic of neurodegenerative and autoimmune diseases today—such as Parkinson's, Alzheimer's, attention deficit disorder (ADD), fibromyalgia and chronic fatigue syndrome, among others. In our first book, *Create a Toxin-Free Body & Home Starting Today,* we describe in greater detail the dangers of heavy metals, especially mercury.

Fructose, which is the natural sugar found in fruit, has also been found to be worse than the sucrose in cane sugar for creating Syndrome X.

Generally, the larger the fish, the more toxic heavy metals it contains; therefore, we recommend avoiding consuming all medium and large-sized fish on a regular basis—tasty as they are.

The Natural Resources Defense Council has a chart on its website: *nrdc.org/health/effects/mercury/calculator/start.asp* where you can calculate the amount of mercury that you are exposed to when you eat different types of fish. This chart also provides recommendations for safe intake levels of various fish.

As a general rule, very small, bony fish, like sardines and anchovies, are safe to eat two to three times per week, as are Alaskan and Norweigan wild salmon that are caught far from the shore. Shellfish, farm-raised fish and most other types of larger wild-caught fish should be eaten only rarely. Shellfish live on the ocean/sea floor and accumulate higher levels of mercury and other heavy metals from our polluted oceans, lakes and waterways than other fish in the same waters.

Farm-raised fish are usually fed pesticide and herbicide-contaminated feed as well as "animal-enhanced protein"—which is basically the discarded remains of slaughtered cows and chickens.

If you eat fish, consider taking a heavy-metal binding supplement such as Zeolite-HP (by NutraMedix: *NutraMedix.com*), or cell-wall-cracked chlorella immediately after eating the fish, to bind the mercury and other metals that get released from the fish into your gut. This will ensure that they get shuttled out of your body instead of absorbed into it.

White Foods

White foods, such as white potatoes, flour, sugar, bread, and pasta are another category of food that will make most of us fat, sick and tired, so we recommend avoiding these foods as much as possible.

White flour can cause celiac disease, gluten sensitivities, gut allergies, and baldness, among other maladies. All white flour is made from wheat, and most wheat is genetically modified. Also, when flour is bleached white, many nutrients are eliminated from it. Consider white flour an essentially nutrient-deficient food.

SUGAR

On average, people in the United States eat 150 pounds of sugar per year. At least half of these people are at a greater risk for heart attacks, stroke, and other serious illnesses. Many of us are also at risk for the much talked about Syndrome X, which is characterized by weight gain (especially in the abdomen); high blood pressure, cholesterol and insulin levels, and an increased risk for diabetes, strokes and heart attacks.

We can avoid and resolve this syndrome by avoiding all sugars and our exposure to plastics. Even the natural sugar found in some fruits and fruit juice, can skyrocket blood sugar levels and create susceptibility to diabetes and weight problems in some people.

The best way to remove plastic from the body is with a far infrared sauna, which removes bisphenol-A (BPA), phthalates and some other types of plastic residue.

High fructose corn syrup may be the most harmful form of sugar. A popular television ad that states that corn syrup is "just another sugar" is misleading. It is a poisonous sugar that harms the body in many ways. It damages artery walls, raises cholesterol, increases diabetes risk, and causes cirrhosis and a fatty liver, among other things. Fructose, which is the natural sugar found in fruit, has also been found to be worse than the sucrose in cane sugar for creating Syndrome X.

Foods Contaminated by Plastic

We all ingest plastics because most of our food is packaged in plastic, which then leeches into our food and beverages. Water bottles, food storage containers and food wrap are the biggest sources of plastic. When this plastic gets into our bodies, it acts as a type of fake estrogen and disrupts our delicate hormonal balance and increases our susceptibility to cancer, sterility, PMS and premature menopause, just to name a few conditions.

Phthalates, which are a type of chemical that comes from plastic, poison insulin receptors on our cells. These receptors enable the cell to receive glucose for energy so phthalates predispose people to insulin resistance, which is the trigger for, and hallmark condition of, Syndrome X.

Bisphenol-A (BPA), a plastic ingredient that is used to line metal food and drink cans, has been linked to birth defects, breast and prostate cancer, and infertility, among other conditions.

Whenever possible, avoid canned food, food stored in plastic and plastic beverage bottles. It's especially important to avoid purchasing moist foods packaged in plastic, such as lunch meat, as these absorb more phthalates and other plastic-derived chemicals from their plastic wrapping than other types of food. Frozen vegetables and fruits that are bagged in plastic also contain small amounts of plastic residue, so it's always better to eat vegetables, fruits and meats fresh.

Most large grocery stores still have butchers that sell meat wrapped in butcher's paper, rather than plastic, so your exposure to plastic will be less if you purchase your meat directly from a butcher rather than from the store shelves.

Most granola and so-called health food snacks sold in health food stores have canola oil added to them, but any food that contains canola is not healthy.

Fortunately, there are a couple of ways that you can remove accumulated plastic from your body. The best way is with a far infrared sauna, which removes bisphenol-A (BPA), phthalates and some other types of plastic residue. Secondly, fiber can sometimes bind to phthalates and other plastic chemicals, and carry them out of the body, but your best option is to do an infrared sauna.

Foods are best stored in glass, steel or ceramic containers, and beverages are best stored in glass bottles.

Hydrogenated Oils and Transfats

Hydrogenated and partially hydrogenated fats, such as transfats, are found in margarine, most shortening products and many cooking oils, as well as in processed and packaged foods. Margarine and other artificial buttery spreads are particularly high in transfats. These fats raise levels of harmful cholesterol and are extremely damaging to the body. Cooking oils with these fats can be identified by the words, "hydrogenated" or "partially-hydrogenated" on their ingredient labels.

Avoid these fats like the plague! They cause obesity, dysfunction and destruction of cells, as well as cell and organelle membranes. Organelles are structures inside the cell that are akin in their functions to the organs of the body. Depending on what type of cell is affected, this dysfunction results in symptoms such as fatigue, brain fog and memory loss. It also results in immune dysfunction, and hampers the cells' ability to produce enzymes and essential proteins for the body. If your body's enzymes are defective, then nothing works, and you can't make neurotransmitters, hormones, digestive enzymes, metabolic enzymes and other structures that produce energy for the cell. Such cellular destruction also results in premature aging.

Other oils that are harmful to the body include soybean, peanut, canola, cottonseed and corn oil. Cold-pressed sunflower, safflower and grape seed oils are okay if they are stored in the refrigerator.

Healthy cell membranes enable the cells to efficiently receive nutrients and expel harmful waste products.

Canola oil, which some people believe to be healthy, is really genetically modified "rape" seed oil and was sold in Canada until several people died from consuming it. After that, the Canadian food industry, through genetic engineering, lowered the amount of the harmful chemical that was found in the rape seed oil and then renamed it canola oil. So while the GMO-rape seed oil is no longer deadly, it isn't healthy either.

Most granola and so-called health food snacks sold in health food stores have canola oil added to them, but any food that contains canola is not healthy. Both canola and peanut oil have very long chain fatty acids that damage cell membranes.

(See Chapter Four, *Foods that Will Make you Healthy and Happy...*, page 70, for a bolded list of healthful nuts and oils.)

Fried Foods

Fried foods, tasty as they are, aren't that good for you either, so we recommend avoiding fried foods whenever possible. Frying causes the healthy fats in food to oxidize, which then generates cell-damaging and DNA-altering free radicals in the body that can lead to cancer, strokes and heart attacks.

Lots of restaurants serve fried foods that contain large amounts of oxidized fats and transfats, so if you are concerned about your exposure to these fats, it's best to eat at high-quality, healthy restaurants, or not order fried food when you go out.

Omega-6 fatty acids are found in most processed and fast foods; cooking oils and nuts, as well as in animal protein, especially animals raised on corn or other types of omega-6 EFA-rich feed.

Eggs are generally good for you, but not if they are fried, scrambled or prepared as an omelet. When you expose the cholesterol in egg yolks to heat and oxygen at the same time, it produces oxycholesterol, which, as we described previously, is a harmful type of cholesterol. So it is best to eat your eggs lightly poached or soft-boiled in the shell. Wait until after the egg is cooked to break its yolk.

Most oils, other than palm kernel or coconut oil, contain unsaturated fatty acids. When healthy unsaturated oil is exposed to oxygen in the air, especially at room temperature or above, the oil can chemically bind to oxygen and become a rancid or oxidized fat. Oxidized fats inflame the arteries and cause heart attacks, strokes and otherwise damage the cells that incorporate those fats into their membranes. Therefore, it is important to keep most oils, except for palm kernel and coconut oil, in the fridge after opening the bottle for the first time.

You'll also want to avoid peanuts, peanut butter and peanut oil. Peanuts contain mold toxins, or mycotoxins, which are produced by fungi. These cause cancer, suppress the immune system, are non-degradable, and accumulate in the tissues over time. Peanut oils have very long chain fatty acids that disrupt the function and activity of every cell in the body. Peanuts provide no net benefits to the body whatsoever! Almond butter is a much better choice than peanut butter.

Too Many Omega-6 Essential Fatty Acid Foods

Omega-6 essential fatty acids (EFAs) and omega-3 EFAs are polyunsaturated fats that support the cardiovascular, reproductive, immune and nervous systems. The human body uses EFAs to manufacture and repair cell membranes. They are called essential fats because the body cannot manufacture them and they must be obtained from foods or dietary supplements. Healthy cell membranes enable the cells to efficiently receive nutrients and expel harmful waste products.

EFAs also support the production of healthy brain and nervous system tissue, and are necessary for making hormones and prostaglandins, the latter of which are fatty molecules that regulate body functions such as heart rate, blood pressure, blood clotting, fertility and inflammation. When the body is deficient in EFAs, its cell membranes become rigid or stiff, which is a sign of aging.

Unfortunately, most of us have too many omega-6 EFAs in our diets. This causes inflammation in the body when these EFAs aren't balanced by the proper amount of omega-3 EFAs. Feed-lot, or conventionally processed beef and caged chickens that are fed corn and other grains have higher amounts of omega-6 EFAs in their meat, which is another good reason to avoid them.

Omega-6 fatty acids are found in most processed and fast foods, cooking oils and nuts, as well as in animal protein, especially animals raised on corn or other types of omega-6 EFA-rich feed.

Most of us need to be vigilant about how many omega-6 EFAs we consume, and restrict the omega-6 EFA foods in our diets, especially the unhealthy sources of omega-6 EFAs. At the same time, most of us could benefit from increasing the amount of omega-3 fatty acids in our diets.

Omega-3 EFAs come from oily fish like sardines, anchovies, salmon and mackerel, and to a lesser extent other ocean fishes. Walnuts, flaxseed oil and chia seeds also contain omega-3 EFAs, but some people's bodies cannot effectively utilize the omega-3 EFAs in plant-based foods because they have to be converted by an enzyme in the body to a usable form. This conversion process is impaired when the person is under stress. Omega-3 EFAs from wild salmon, sardines, anchovies and fish oil supplements are therefore a better source of this nutrient.

ARTIFICIAL SWEETENERS

All artificial sweeteners, no matter their caloric content, damage the brain and nervous system and increase cancer risk. Splenda (sucralose), Sweet'N Low (saccharin), Equal and Nutrasweet (aspartame) are among the worst offenders. The herbal sweetener stevia is an acceptable alternative to these artificial sweeteners as long as it is in a liquid form, as many of the filler ingredients used in powdered stevia are unhealthy.

Possibly the best place to buy food is directly from your local organic farmer.

As depressing as all of this information may seem, it's impossible to provide guidelines for eating healthy food without mentioning the toxicity of our food supply and how to avoid toxic foods. If we want to be healthy and live long we need to eat clean food. It's that simple.

CHAPTER FOUR

Foods that Will Make You Healthy, Happy, Energetic and Trim

After reading Chapter Three, *Foods That Make Everyone Sick, Fat and Tired,* you may be wondering if any of the foods that line supermarket shelves are healthy anymore. The answer is yes! You just need a few simple rules for identifying them.

The first rule of thumb when looking for healthy food is to choose foods that are in as natural a state as possible. Such foods promote health and emotional well-being, and are readily digested by the body. Just as important, choose clean, nutrient-dense foods, which are best found at your local health food store, organic farmers' market or local organic farm.

Some grocers have an organic food section, but most grocery stores in the US don't carry enough organic food to meet all of the body's needs. Also, organic food may be more expensive in conventional supermarkets than in health food stores. Possibly the best place to buy food is directly from your local organic farmer. We encourage this for several reasons.

Fortunately, by eating organic food, we can still obtain healthy food in today's world. While there is no such thing as a one-size-fits-all diet, there are some categories and types of foods that most of us will respond well to, which promote health, vitality and well-being.

First, the fruits and vegetables that come from local farms are likely to have a higher nutritional content than those which come from other states or countries, because they aren't picked prior to maturity and shipped across many miles. Most fruits and vegetables, when they must be shipped thousands of miles, are picked early so that they don't become overripe in transit. This causes them to have an inferior nutrient content than produce that is allowed to ripen to maturity.

Also, small organic farmers often grow their food in soil that is superior in quality and mineral content to that of large industrialized farms, and their livestock tend to be raised under more humane conditions than animals on large factory farms.

Another nice benefit of buying from a local farm is that you can often get to know your local farmers and see for yourself how the food is being produced, rather than relying on product labels to determine whether you are buying quality food.

Buying from local farmers also discourages the further development of large-scale industrial or factory farming practices, since, through your purchases, you support local farming. It also saves on waste, fuel costs and energy (since the food doesn't have to travel a long distance), and benefits the environment and humanity in other ways.

For more information about the differences between large-scale, industrialized organic farming and true organic farming, and the advantages of purchasing food from a local organic farm or farmers' market instead of the supermarket, we highly recommend reading Michael Pollan's award-winning book, *The Omnivore's Dilemma.* His pocket-sized book, *Food Rules,* is another excellent resource on healthy eating because it describes in simple terms how to eat well without having to follow a complex dietary protocol.

The basic premise of *Food Rules*—which we advocate in this book as well—is to eat real food, such as vegetables, fruits, whole grains, fish, and meat—and avoid what Michael calls "edible food-like substances." *Food Rules,* which contains sixty-four short rules for eating well, provides tidbits of common sense, yet valuable information that can help most of us who are confused by what's healthy and what's not in the supermarket, to make wise food choices.

For example, Pollan advocates not eating anything that your great-grandmother wouldn't recognize as food, because our ancestors had no choice but to consume natural food!

He also suggests not eating products that contain more than five ingredients, or ingredients that you can't pronounce, and encourages shopping around the perimeter of the supermarket,

Most of us feel and function at our best when our daily meals include modest palm-sized portions of healthy animal protein.

since that is where you are most likely to find real food such as produce and fresh animal protein.

Fortunately, we can obtain healthy organic food in today's world. While there is no such thing as a one-size-fits-all diet, there are some categories and types of foods that most of us will respond well to, which promote health, vitality and well-being. In the following sections, we describe these.

Before you run out and purchase any of these foods, however, we recommend reading this book through to the end, because you may find that some of the types of food that we are about to describe—healthy as they are!—would be better suited to people with a different biochemistry or body type than yours.

In Part Two we'll show you how to choose foods that fit your specific body type, but first, we want to provide some general tips on how to select healthy categories of food.

Organic Vegetables

Just about every diet book on the market advocates eating vegetables. And in fact, veggies are good for most everyone, with few exceptions. They are a rich source of carbohydrates, which provide energy to the cells. Most are rich in beta-carotene (which is converted by the body into Vitamin A), B-vitamins, Vitamins C, K and dietary minerals such as calcium, magnesium, potassium, and iron. They also contain a variety of yet to be identified trace nutrients that are essential for health, and which you cannot obtain from supplements. This is one reason why we can't just get all of our nutrients from vitamins.

Additionally, vegetables contain high levels of antioxidants, which help the body to scavenge DNA-damaging free radical chemicals in the bloodstream that can lead to cellular destruction, inflammation, obesity and cancer. Some also have antibacterial, antifungal and antiviral properties, and as such, help the body to ward off infections. Many vegetables also contain fiber, which is necessary for healthy gastrointestinal function. Vegetables protect the body against a wide variety of illnesses and health conditions, including cancer, diabetes, and kidney stones.

If your body likes animal protein—and most people's do—then we advocate including one to four servings of meat into your daily meals and snacks.

Non-starchy vegetables, which include green veggies such as lettuces, spinach, bok-choy, arugula, kale, endive, parsley, asparagus, broccoli, zucchini, green beans and Brussels sprouts, as well as cabbage, summer squash, onions and garlic, are especially well-tolerated by a majority of people.

While nightshade vegetables are nutrient-rich, they cause inflammation in some people. Common nightshade vegetables include white potatoes, tomatoes, eggplant and peppers (hot and sweet). These veggies contain a substance called alkaloids that can negatively impact nerve, muscle and digestive function, and cause inflammation, especially in people with certain chronic health conditions, such as fibromyalgia, chronic fatigue syndrome, Lyme disease, arthritis, colitis, and autoimmune disease.

High-glycemic vegetables, such as carrots and beets, are likewise problematic for some people. In general, however, organic vegetables are among the most nutritious, health-promoting foods we can eat. Most people will want to include multiple servings of any of the following into their daily diet:

- Artichoke
- Arugula
- Bok choy
- Broccoli
- Brussels sprouts
- Cabbage
- Celery
- Collard greens
- Cucumbers
- Garlic
- Green onions
- Endive
- Kale
- Leeks

- Lettuce
- Mustard greens
- Onions
- Parsley
- Radish
- Scallions
- Seaweed
- Spinach
- Sprouts
- String beans
- Summer squash
- Swiss Chard
- Watercress
- Zucchini

If you don't have a serious health condition, especially chronic fatigue syndrome, fibromyalgia, Candida, hypoglycemia or blood-sugar imbalance problems, you may also be able to add some starchy and nightshade vegetables to this list, including:

- Beet (roots)
- Bell (and other peppers)
- Carrots
- Eggplant
- Mushrooms
- Parsnips (roots)

- Red potatoes
- Sweet potatoes
- Tomatoes
- Winter squash/pumpkin
- Yams
- Yucca

CLEAN, ORGANIC ANIMAL PROTEIN

Clean, organic animal protein should be an important staple of most people's diets. Most of us feel and function at our best when our daily meals include modest palm-sized portions of healthy animal protein, including free-range chicken and eggs; grass-fed, non-GMO beef; wild salmon, sardines, anchovies and other small fish; lamb, ostrich, turkey, Cornish game hen, buffalo, elk, bison and other game meat.

Indeed, if your body welcomes animal protein—and most people's bodies do—then we advocate including 1-4 servings of meat into your daily meals and snacks. The number of servings of animal protein that you need will depend upon your metabolic type and other factors. Metabolic typing is described in Part Two.

The only types of protein that we don't advocate eating on a regular basis are shellfish and pork. Shellfish are "bottom dwellers"—fish that are known for filtering out toxins from the ocean, and which therefore accumulate a much higher content of heavy metals and other toxins than most bony fish. Both pork and shellfish are unclean meats. Pigs eat most everything, even dead animals, and their meat often contains parasites, which can then infect your body.

Besides the fact that they are cleaner, free-range animals are preferable to conventionally processed animals because their meat contains more health-promoting omega-3 essential fatty acids than conventionally processed meat. This is because their diets contain a greater diversity of healthy foods, and they therefore have more micro-nutrients concentrated into their meat.

> Organic nuts and seeds (except for peanuts) are an important source of healthy fat and protein for most of us and are used by our bodies as building blocks for hormones, organs and other tissue.

The body uses omega-3 acids to make brain tissue and cell membranes. The most prevalent fatty acid in the brain is called DHA. It is found in free-range animals as well as in fish, and is important for normal brain function. If you don't eat much animal protein, you'll want to take DHA as a supplement, to ensure that your brain gets the nutrition that it needs.

Fish

Certain fish are healthy and provide essential fatty acids to the body, which, as we previously mentioned, are important for reducing inflammation and are a key component in the structure and function of all cell membranes and fatty tissues in the body, especially the brain.

We advocate eating only small, wild-caught bony fish, and taking a toxin-binding supplement whenever you eat any kind of fish, to keep any heavy metals from the fish from binding to your tissues and organs. Some people don't like anchovies or sardines, but they can be made tastier if they are eaten as part of a salad or spiced up with mustard or olive oil and sea salt.

ORGANIC FRUITS

Organic fruits are rich in vitamins, minerals, micronutrients, fiber and antioxidants, and provide energy and health to the body in a variety of ways. Because of their high vitamin content, particularly Vitamin C, most fruits boost the immune system. The antioxidants in fruit help to remove DNA-damaging free radicals from the body that lead to cancer and aging; lower unhealthy cholesterol, promote healthy digestion and protect the body against a multitude of ailments, from hair and memory loss and wrinkled skin, to age-related macular degeneration (ARMD of the retina in the eyes); Alzheimer's and heart disease; colon cancers, weak bones, and more.

Even people who don't feel bad after eating a slice of bread or bowl of pasta are likely to feel more energetic and fare better on a diet of tasty, healthy non-gluten grains, such as quinoa, amaranth, millet, spelt and brown rice.

Most people can consume at least a modest amount of fruit, and doing so contributes to a healthy body and physique. Some people shouldn't eat fruits that contain high amounts of natural sugar, such as bananas, papayas, grapes and melons, and will feel better if they stick to fruits with a lower natural sugar content, such as avocados, berries, grapefruit, lemon, and green apples.

Most people should also avoid fruit juice, since it causes blood sugar spikes that can lead to hypoglycemia, inflammation and insulin resistance. In Part Two, Chapter Five, *Your Current Health Condition,* we describe the types of fruit that people with different health conditions should eat and which they should avoid.

Organic Nuts and Seeds

Organic nuts and seeds (except for peanuts and "rape" seeds) are an important source of healthy fat and protein for most of us and are used by our bodies as building blocks for hormones, organs and other tissue.

Most nuts and seeds contain high amounts of fiber, as well as vitamins and minerals, especially Vitamin E, selenium, calcium, magnesium, potassium, copper, phosphorus, iron and beta-carotene. Studies have shown nuts to protect against cardiovascular disease, and when eaten in moderation, they are a healthful replacement for sugary snacks.

Some of the most nutrient-rich nuts and seeds include organic walnuts, almonds, Brazil nuts, pine nuts, and pecans;

flaxseed and sunflower, pumpkin, and sesame seeds, as well as nut and seed butters that are made from these nuts and which don't contain sugar or other additives.

We recommend consuming no more than a couple of handfuls daily of nuts or seeds, as they are calorie-dense and can easily cause weight gain. Also, most nuts and seeds contain higher levels of omega-6 EFAs than omega-3 EFAs, and an imbalance of omega-3 and omega-6 fatty acids in the body causes inflammation, which can lead to weight gain and other health problems. Walnuts, chia seeds and flaxseeds contain more healthy ratios of omega-3 to omega-6 fats compared to other nuts and seeds, and may therefore be a better choice than some of the others.

Non-Gluten Grains and Legumes

Have you ever noticed how many people nowadays are allergic to gluten, which is found principally in wheat, but also in other grains and other types of products, such as condiments and dressings? This is partly because condiments, dressings, breads and other grain products contain massive amounts of the stuff nowadays, which the body isn't designed to digest. Years ago, bread was good for you. But now, many people are gluten-intolerant due to the overabundance of gluten in the food supply, especially in genetically modified wheat.

> Cow's milk products, organic or not, are generally not well-suited to humans. But most of us will reap some health benefits from organic goat and sheep milk products, especially cheese, kefir and yogurt.

Fortunately, most people can still tolerate modest amounts of gluten grains, but as a general rule, more of us than not will do better eating less of this type of food than the others that we've mentioned so far.

Even people who don't feel bad after eating a slice of bread or bowl of pasta are likely to feel more energetic and fare better on a diet of tasty, healthy non-gluten grains, such as quinoa, amaranth, millet, spelt and brown rice.

Amaranth, which was originally cultivated by the Aztec people of Mexico, is a grain that contains all of the amino acids or protein building blocks that are essential for human health. Quinoa, which was originally cultivated by the Inca people of South America, is especially healthful. It isn't a true grain, but rather, a seed that also contains all of the essential amino acids, as well as higher levels of protein than any other grain or seed.

Fortunately, most health food stores sell flours, pastas, breads and other grain products made from a variety of non-gluten grains, and which are just as tasty as gluten-containing grains.

Legumes, such as lima, black, kidney and other types of beans; black-eyed peas, lentils, and chickpeas, are also healthy foods for most of us, but, like grains, they are best consumed in moderation. People with a certain metabolic type can eat legumes and grains daily, and in Part Two of this book, we describe the concept of metabolic typing and how to determine your metabolic type, which can be used as a tool for further refining your diet.

Weston Price, an early 1900s dentist, traveled the globe and found that the societies that had the best physical and dental health were those that never consumed grains. Fortunately, however, grains can be healthful for people with certain metabolic types, especially when they are eaten in moderation.

Organic Goat/Sheep Milk Cheese

While cow's milk products, organic or not, are generally not well suited to humans, most of us will reap some health benefits from organic goat and sheep milk products, especially cheese, kefir and yogurt. These can be healthful sources of protein and are a tasty addition to most of our diets.

Probiotic supplements and yogurt contain, at most, a dozen types of bacteria that the gut needs for optimal wellness, but fermented foods, like kimchi and sauerkraut, can provide up to several hundred species.

In general, most of us will function better on a diet that includes greater amounts of fruits, vegetables and meats, and lesser amounts of grains, legumes or milk products, but again, everyone is different, and in Part Two, we help you to decide how and what to eat, according to your individual biochemistry.

Plain Organic Yogurt and Other Probiotic Foods

Many brands and types of yogurt fill our grocery store shelves, but our bodies tolerate few of these without going into a tailspin of inflammation. Most yogurts, even those which are organic, low-fat, and labeled "natural" contain real or artificial sweeteners and an abundance of unhealthy chemicals to preserve them, are made from cow's milk, and have been stripped of valuable nutrients because they are pasteurized and homogenized.

Nonetheless, yogurt can be a valuable source of protein, as well as minerals such as magnesium and calcium, and immune-enhancing probiotics, or immune-supportive bacteria, which we need for a healthy gastrointestinal tract and immune system. In most cases, these bacteria are stripped from the yogurt during pasteurization and replenished afterwards, but your body will still derive some benefit from them.

Raw yogurt is the most health promoting, because it isn't pasteurized and therefore contains all of its original beneficial bacteria and enzymes. Raw yogurt isn't sold in grocery stores, however—you'll need to make it yourself or obtain it from a raw dairy farm.

If you do an Internet search and input the term "raw dairy farm" into the search engine box, along with your city and/or state, you are likely to find farms in your area that sell raw dairy products. Similarly, instructions for how to make homemade yogurt can easily be found on the Internet on websites such as: *MakeYourOwnYogurt.com*.

Finally, while yogurt is somewhat nutritious, it also increases mucus production in the respiratory and GI tracts, as well as the lymphatic system. Mucus can cause sinus infections, hinder toxin removal through the lymphatic system, impair nutrient absorption in the gut, and encourage the growth of pathogens in the sinuses that can then lead to systemic infections. For these reasons, most of us should consume yogurt only in moderation.

Kimchi

Kimchi is a flavorful and healthy fermented Korean food that can replenish the gut with immune-supportive friendly bacteria when it gets depleted by stress and the garbage that's found in the conventional food supply, particularly antibiotics.

Healthy oils and fats are integral to a healthy diet. Healthy oils and fats include coconut, palm kernel, MCT, almond, walnut, flaxseed, macadamia and olive oils; ghee (clarified butter) and organic butter, as well as nuts of all kinds (except peanuts).

A healthy human gut has approximately 500 to 1,000 types of friendly bacteria. People who have taken antibiotics or eaten conventionally processed beef, however, might only have a few dozen, since antibiotics strip the gut of these bacteria. These bacteria are our bodies' first line of defense against viruses, bacteria, parasites and other pathogens, which enter our gut through our food and drink. If you don't have enough friendly bacteria in your gastro-intestinal tract, you become more susceptible to infections and illness, and your body won't process nutrients as effectively.

Probiotic supplements and yogurt contain, at most, a dozen types of bacteria that the gut needs for optimal wellness, but fermented foods, like kimchi and sauerkraut, can provide up to several hundred species! For that reason, we highly recommend including ample amounts of these foods into your diet. You can make kimchi yourself, and starter kits are sold at most health food stores. You can also buy ready-made kimchi.

Sprouted Foods

Sprouting is the practice of germinating seeds to be eaten raw or cooked. Sprouted foods are a valuable addition to any dietary regimen, because they are rich in bio-available vitamins, minerals, amino acids, proteins and phytochemicals. Many seeds can be sprouted, whether they come from beans, nuts, seeds, or even cruciferous vegetables.

Sea salt is incredibly nutritious for most. The best salt to use is Himalayan salt, which is dug out of the ground in the Himalayan mountains and originates from a prehistoric sea bed.

For the sprouting process, seeds are soaked in water for anywhere from 20 minutes to 12 hours, then placed in a sprouting vessel, such as a jar covered with a nylon or other cloth rim, for three to five days.

During this time, the metabolic activity of the seeds increases and their protein, starch and lipids (fats) are broken down into simple compounds by enzymes that are used to make new compounds. The resultant compounds are rich in nutrients, including vitamins, minerals, proteins and even essential fatty acids, depending on the seed that you use.

Sprouts are incredibly nutritious. Studies have shown some sprouted foods to contain up to fifteen times the amount of nutrients found in the original food. Sprouts are also referred to as pre-digested food because the food's macronutrients are broken down during the sprouting process. This makes them easier to digest than the original seed, bean, nut or grain.

Sprouted foods also contain higher amounts of enzymes than unsprouted foods, which also makes them more digestible. Sprouted foods are therefore one great way to ensure that you are getting all of the nutrients that you need into your diet. Don't cook sprouted foods or you will remove many of the beneficial nutrients that were activated during the sprouting process.

Healthy Oils and Fats

Healthy oils and fats are integral to a healthy diet. Healthy oils and fats include coconut, palm kernel, MCT, almond, walnut, flaxseed, macadamia and olive oils; ghee (clarified butter) and organic butter, as well as nuts of all kinds (except peanuts).

These are important for brain function, healthy cell membranes and for the formation of fats used to make hormones, which carry messages from glands to cells within tissues or organs of the body. Hormones also maintain chemical levels in the bloodstream to help achieve homeostasis or a state of balance within the body.

The healthiest oil for cooking is palm kernel oil. This is a fully saturated oil that, when heated, doesn't hydrogenate and form transfats, or become rancid and oxidize. Coconut and MCT oil are also very healthy cooking oils.

> Nowadays, it is essential to use a reverse osmosis or carbon block water filter for all of your drinking and bathing water.

SPICES AND SAUCES

Spices and sauces give food their desirable flavor. Most have antioxidant, anti-inflammatory and antimicrobial properties— that is, they fight against bad bacteria—and are therefore good for the body, as well as delicious. You can enhance your health and the taste of foods by preparing foods with a variety of spices besides salt. Some spices have specific health benefits. For example, cinnamon balances blood sugar, and cilantro and garlic bind heavy metals.

The best salt to use is Himalayan salt, which is dug out of the ground in the Himalayan mountains and originates from a prehistoric sea bed. There are no environmental pollutants in this salt as you might find in other salts.

HEALTHY SWEETENERS

Stevia is an herb that is made from the stevia plant, which is also called honey leaf. It can be used to sweeten beverages, desserts and other foods. It is thought by some people to be sweeter than sugar and is an excellent alternative to sugar. So if you eat very little sugar, four drops of stevia extract might seem like the equivalent of one teaspoon of sugar to your taste buds. If your taste buds have been desensitized by lots of sugar, however, you might need 12 drops to experience the same amount of sweetness.

Chinese monk fruit is another sweetener that is a good substitute for sugar and which is becoming increasingly available in health food stores and at online retailers.

Nutritious Cooking Flours

Organic nut, bean and gluten-free grain flours are better choices of baking flours than white or wheat flours. Almond flour is the most nutritious type of flour to bake with, due to its low starch and sugar content, and is a healthy source of flour if you aren't allergic to almonds. Health food stores carry these types of flour, but you can find a wider variety on the Internet.

Clean Water and Other Healthy Beverages

Finally, just as it is important to consume natural, organic, clean food, it is also essential to drink clean water. Unfortunately, just as our food supply has become polluted, so most all tap water nowadays is contaminated by fluoride, chlorine, asbestos, plastics, pesticides, antibiotics, pharmaceutical drugs, heavy metals and other industrial contaminants. Microorganisms, including parasites and viruses, are also prevalent in tap water.

Nowadays, it is essential to use a reverse osmosis or carbon block water filter for all of your drinking and bathing water, if you want to avoid bodily contamination by these pollutants.

If you can't afford a good water filter, some health food stores sell bottled water that has been purified via reverse osmosis, or you can have purified water delivered to your home in five gallon bottles.

People gain weight not only because they eat lots of contaminated food, harmful fats, sugars or excessive amounts of starchy carbohydrates, but also because they eat foods that are wrong for their body type, and in the wrong amounts.

Make sure to purchase water in glass bottles or phthalate and BPA-free plastic bottles. BPA-free plastic is the only type of plastic that won't leech into the water. Reverse osmosis water is generally sold in the supermarket in one, three and five gallon containers.

Some people prefer to consume distilled water but distillers use up a lot of electrical energy when producing water, so it may be more expensive over the long run to drink distilled water than to purchase a carbon block or reverse osmosis filter for your tap.

If you purchase a water distiller or reverse osmosis filter for your home, it's a good idea to drink the water right after you fill your glass with it. Otherwise, carbon dioxide gas from the air will spontaneously dissolve into the water and make it acidic. Alternatively, you can add trace minerals to the distilled or reverse osmosis water soon after it is made. This will prevent the water from taking up the carbon dioxide as easily.

One disadvantage of carbon block filters is that they remove increasingly fewer contaminants over time, as the carbon gets used up. Some also remove a wider variety of pollutants than others, so it pays to shop around to find a good one. One brand that we highly recommend is Multipure, which removes many types of organic and inorganic pollutants. For a complete list of contaminants that these filters remove, visit: *Multipure.com/mpscience.*

Other beverages that are healthy to drink include: organic herbal tea that has been proven to be free of pesticides, mold and other contaminants; kombucha that contains no sugar or other artificial additives, and vegetable juice that is also additive-free. Many so-called health drinks such as kombucha and fruit juice contain lots of natural or added sugar and harmful additives, so it's important to choose only those drinks that don't contain these sugars and additives.

Part Two

Individualizing Your Diet

As Joe strode across the college campus, weakness swept through his legs. His belly rumbled and head throbbed. The rice and bean salad that he had eaten for lunch wasn't holding him. Once again, he wondered if the vegan diet that Dr. Allen had put him on was such a great idea. He constantly felt his energy tanking by the time he attended his last class at 3 PM, so that he often arrived home shaky and irritable. Usually, he kept some nuts or granola bars in his pocket to stop the mid-afternoon blood sugar drop, but today he'd forgotten. Maybe it was because they didn't always seem to be sufficient, anyway.

But he had wanted to follow Dr. Allen's strict orders to avoid animal protein, since he now had leukemia, and according to Dr. Allen, meat is acidic and cancers are known to flourish in an acidic environment. Never mind that Joe was anemic and a pH test had shown him to be excessively alkaline. Besides, Dr. Allen had said, many studies had proven that people with cancer who eat vegetarian diets survive longer than those who don't.

Joe wanted to be well, but he no longer felt on top of the world. Instead, he was weak, tired and irritable—but not from school, the cancer or his holistic medical treatments.

Once home, Joe went to his room to lie down, but paused first in front of the mirror before his bed. His face and lips were pale, and his jeans had become baggy. Something wasn't right.

Confused, he went to his doctor, who told him that of course he felt badly—after all, he had cancer!

Joe, skeptical of his doctor's words, on a hunch, began to eat steak, hamburgers and chicken again, and within a few days, the color returned to his face, his energy increased, and he became stronger and more upbeat again.

In time, he learned that his body thrived on meat and other heavy foods, and the heavier the food—the better. So when he had limited his diet to vegetables, fruits, legumes and grains, he didn't do well. But once he began eating meat again, his energy and vitality returned, and with that, his ability to heal from the cancer.

Joe's story illustrates the profound truth that we are all unique and require different foods to be well. Some people with cancer may indeed do better on a vegetarian diet, but as you will find in Part Two of this book, some doctors have found their cancer patients to do better on a diet that includes regular portions of animal protein, of all types. There is no such thing as one-size-fits all when it comes to our bodies!

CHAPTER FIVE

Customizing Your Diet with Foods that Fit Your Biochemistry and Body Type

By now we hope that you have a better idea about the categories and types of foods that are wellness-promoting, and how to choose clean, natural and uncontaminated foods that will help you to feel and look your best.

When figuring out the foods that best fit your body type and biochemistry, it's important to determine, first and foremost, whether you have any food allergies.

We suggest using the guidelines in Part One as a baseline for selecting healthy foods for your diet, and the guidelines in this section to tailor a food plan to your body's unique needs. By following these guidelines, you are likely to not only feel better, but also attain your ideal weight more easily.

People gain weight not only because they eat lots of contaminated food, harmful fats, sugars or excessive amounts of starchy carbohydrates, but also because they eat foods that are wrong for their body type, and in the wrong amounts.

By determining the types of foods that best fit your body's needs, and in the correct proportions, you can lose weight, without having to pay too much attention to the caloric content of foods. It is a myth that weight loss is all about how much fat or how many calories you consume. There are cultures around the world that eat more fat than we in the US but who are on the average thinner than we are.

Generally, the foods that are the most weight-gain-producing are those that contain sugar—natural or synthetic. We in the US consume more sugary and starch-laden foods than most other countries, which is one reason for the obesity epidemic in this nation. Common foods in our diet, such as French fried potatoes, refined wheat flour products, white bread, pasta and other foods made from refined sugar, all lead to weight gain. Even starch-laden vegetables drive more insulin into the cells than non-starchy ones and can cause weight gain when eaten in excess.

While eating too much can produce tiredness, you aren't supposed to be fatigued after you eat!

Also, when you eat foods that are wrong for your particular body type, it can lead to weight gain. Some foods will make one person with a certain metabolic type fat, but another person with a different metabolic type thin.

Finally, allergenic foods and contaminated foods cause weight gain. Corn and corn byproducts are especially harmful—corn syrup and starch are among the worst offenders. These cause inflammation that leads to weight gain. Phthalates and other types of plastic chemicals cause estrogen dominance, which also leads to fat storage.

SIX FACTORS TO CONSIDER WHEN CUSTOM-TAILORING A DIET PLAN

When determining the foods that will best fit a unique you, you should take into account six principal factors, including:

1. Any food allergies/sensitivities and how you feel after eating different foods

2. Your current health condition and any health problems/illnesses

3. How a particular food affects your tissue pH (acid/alkaline balance)

4. Your metabolic type

5. Your gut health and stomach acid levels

6. Food lectins

FOOD ALLERGIES AND SENSITIVITIES

When figuring out the foods that best fit your body type and biochemistry, it's important to determine, first and foremost, whether you have any food allergies. Most people nowadays have one or more food allergies, due to the toxicity of our food supply. Most of us no longer absorb and assimilate food as effectively as we used to, and no longer react positively to as many foods as before because so many are contaminated.

You may associate food allergies with hives, sneezing or some other obvious allergy symptom. But did you know that tiredness after eating, a fast heart rate, headaches, brain fog, muscle or joint aches and digestive problems are other clues that your body just ate something that it didn't like?

Avoiding allergenic foods is essential for wellness, because if you eat something that your body doesn't like, it will cause an inflammatory response that over time will weaken your immune system and cause all kinds of symptoms. If you already have a health condition, avoiding allergenic foods is essential if you want to recover from that condition.

Allergenic foods cause inflammation, which damages cells, weakens the body and sets it up for disease.

There are two inexpensive ways to test for food allergies. You can do these easy tests from home and figure out for yourself which foods you are allergic or sensitive to.

First, if you are tired or fatigued after you eat, this may be a sign that you ate an allergenic food, although not everyone recognizes tiredness as such—they simply assume that they ate too much! While eating too much can produce tiredness, you aren't supposed to be fatigued after you eat. The tryptophan in turkey might make you a little sleepy but foods shouldn't bring on excessive tiredness.

So if you ate a normal sized meal and became fatigued afterward, chances are you ate something that you were sensitive or allergic to. Sometimes, people with moderately-severe or severe chronic fatigue will be tired after eating because their energy reserve is so low that even eating a meal causes them to use up more energy than they have to spare, but in general, we should have more energy after we eat—not less.

Sometimes symptoms that result from food allergies and sensitivities can have a delayed onset, and may not appear until many hours, or even a day or two, after you ate the food. The inflammatory immune response that is caused by an allergic reaction may also last for days after exposure to the offending food.

For this reason, when determining food allergies, it's a good idea to eliminate all foods from your diet that you suspect to be allergenic, and avoid consuming them for an extended period of time (perhaps a month or two). Then you can slowly re-introduce them back into your diet, one food at a time every three days, and discern specifically which ones are causing you problems, based on your reaction to each.

The Coca pulse test is another simple way to check for food allergies. To do this, sit in a chair and relax for five minutes immediately prior to eating a meal. Then check your pulse rate. Eat, and then take your pulse again fifteen minutes after the meal. Make sure to remain rested after you eat so that your pulse doesn't get elevated by activity. Also, avoid distressing conversation or TV shows such as the news during or immediately following the meal, while you are waiting to recheck your pulse.

If your pulse rate after the meal is at least 15 beats per minute faster than your pulse before the meal, you may have eaten one or more foods that you are allergic to. If your pulse rate is 10 to 14 beats per minute faster, it is likely that you ate at least one allergenic food. If your pulse rate increases less than 10 beats per minute, it is unlikely that you ate any foods that you were allergic to.

> Don't get caught up in the tyranny of the should's; the mentality that you should eat certain foods because they are supposed to be good for you—or so says society and a thousand diet books!

If you ate lots of different foods during the meal, it will be hard to discern which foods you were allergic to. But if you ate a simple meal consisting of just a few foods, then over the following three days, you could eat each one of those foods separately and take your pulse again to determine which one(s) you were allergic to.

This test doesn't work for nightshade veggies. To determine whether you have an allergy to these foods, leave them out of your normal diet for a few weeks and take note of any differences in how you feel.

FOOD SENSITIVITIES AND INFLAMMATION

Allergenic foods cause inflammation, which damages cells, weakens the body and sets it up for disease. Pain, fatigue, depression, brain fog, and a whole host of other symptoms are triggered by inflammation, as well as weight gain, which is why it's important to avoid inflammatory foods. This is especially important if you are recovering from a serious health condition. Your immune system will be able to fight for you more effectively if you remove all allergenic foods from your diet.

Sugar is one of the worst inflammatory foods. Studies have shown that the average American eats approximately one pound of sugar per pound of body weight per year. Sugar and starches stimulate insulin release, which causes inflammation in the blood vessels and joints, and arthritic symptoms.

Perhaps even worse, insulin receptors, which help to shuttle glucose into the cell for energy production, become de-sensitized by excessive sugar intake, which then results in Syndrome X, a condition that can lead to strokes, high blood pressure, obesity, heart attacks, diabetes, arthritis, and other illnesses. Syndrome X is now estimated to affect half of the adult US population, due in part to the poor quality of our food supply and our diets.

Most of us have at least one symptom—muscle pain, tiredness, brain fog, headaches, gut problems, insomnia, depression, anxiety, or joint pain, just to name a few—as a result of eating the wrong foods, but we don't always attribute our symptoms to our poor diets.

Inflammation is also triggered by contaminated GMO food and arachidonic acid, the latter of which is found in high amounts in peanuts and feedlot beef, so it goes without saying that these types of food should be avoided.

Some people have a genetic defect that prevents them from detoxifying solanine from their bodies. Solanine is a natural poison found in nightshade vegetables such as tomatoes, potatoes, eggplant and peppers. People with this problem will develop inflammation if they eat solanine-containing foods. You can determine whether you have problems detoxifying solanine by removing nightshade vegetables from your diet for a few weeks and observing any changes in how you feel.

How Does the Food Make You Feel?

It's amazing how many of us eat without paying attention to whether food makes us tired or grumpy—or causes other uncomfortable symptoms. Yet paying attention to how you feel after a meal is a main key to discovering the foods that are right for you, and the ones that are not.

Again, you're supposed to feel good after you eat—always! Do you feel more energetic? Do you have less pain? Are you in a better mood? If you ate the right stuff, you should feel better overall.

Don't get caught up in the tyranny of the should's; the mentality that you should eat certain foods because they are supposed to be good for you—or so says society and a thousand diet books! Eat what makes your body feel right, not what the latest diet book tells you is good for you.

Now, if you just ate some pasta because your blood sugar tanked and you became shaky and tired, and you felt more stable after eating the pasta, it doesn't necessarily mean that the pasta was good for you. If you felt better in one way (i.e. your mood and shakiness stabilized) but worse in another (you became exhausted after the meal), then chances are, what you gave your body wasn't good for it.

The proportions of food that you eat matter, too. Protein, carbohydrate and fat portions must all be balanced. Some people need more protein from animal sources while others may need more fatty or carbohydrate foods, and any imbalance of these in a meal can cause you to feel either dissatisfied or less than your best.

It's best to experiment with food portions to determine how much of each type of food that you need. Generally, most people eat too many grains—breads, cereals, rice, pasta, and the like, and too few non-starchy veggies, healthy fats or animal protein products. Depending on your constitution and metabolic characteristics, you may need less of one or more of the other.

YOUR CURRENT HEALTH CONDITION

Few adults nowadays, even young adults, feel really great, due in part to our contaminated and nutrient-depleted food supply, as well as our hectic lifestyles and toxic environment. Most of us have at least one symptom—muscle pain, tiredness, brain fog, headaches, gut problems, insomnia, depression, anxiety, or joint pain, just to name a few—as a result of eating the wrong foods, but we don't always attribute our symptoms to our poor diets. Yet if we can discover and begin eating the foods that are the best fit for our bodies, we will often see these symptoms disappear.

If you already have a health condition or illness, it's essential that you formulate a food plan that first and foremost takes into account that condition. In the following sections we describe seventeen of the most common chronic health conditions that people in the industrialized world suffer from—and then suggest foods to eat and foods to avoid if you have any one of these conditions.

To discover whether you have mold toxicity, we recommend consulting Dr. Ritchie Shoemaker's books: *Mold Warriors* and *Surviving Mold: Life in the Era of Dangerous Buildings.*

By following these guidelines, we believe that you will feel better, experience fewer symptoms, and maybe even attain remission from the condition that afflicts you.

CHAPTER SIX

Food Guidelines for Seventeen Different Health Conditions

1. FUNGAL INFECTIONS

Many people nowadays have yeast infections such as Candida or some other type of fungal overgrowth in their bodies, due to the abundance of sugar and antibiotics in our food supply. We also breathe in fungi and mold, which can lead to systemic infections.

Many diet books on Candida have already been written, so here we simply provide some basic guidelines for you to follow if you know that you have Candida, mold or other type of fungal infection. You should follow this diet for only as long as you have the fungal infection, as, once the infection is gone, you are likely to fare better on a diet that's based on your metabolic type. Metabolic typing is described in Chapter Seven, *Food Combining Techniques for Optimal Digestion.*

Symptoms of Candida and other fungal infections can overlap with symptoms of other health conditions; therefore, we recommend doing a saliva or blood test to determine whether you have a fungal infection. One simple, do-it-yourself saliva test for Candida can be found at the National Candida Center website: *NationalCandidaCenter.com/candida-self-exams/*.

Common symptoms of Candida and other yeast infections include, but aren't limited to: intense cravings for sugar, sweets and breads; brain fog, anxiety, mood swings, fatigue, headaches, and skin infections such as eczema, psoriasis and acne. A complete list of symptoms can be found on the National Candida Center website: *NationalCandidaCenter.com*.

Fungi are dangerous because they can produce chemical toxins (mycotoxins) which poison the body. They also invade and damage the tissues and organs.

If you are actively battling cancer, the fungal diet is a very good diet for you to follow as well, at least for as long as you are treating the cancer, since cancer feeds on sugars of all kinds—fruit sugar, as well as the glucose that the body makes from grains and other starchy foods.

Environmental mycotoxin inhalation is another serious fungal-related condition. Mycotoxins are mold toxins that accumulate in the body and which are fat-soluble. They lead to cancer, immune system suppression, chronic fatigue syndrome, and other serious conditions. The body doesn't have innate mechanisms to detoxify mycotoxins, so it's important to remove them with toxin binders and far infrared saunas.

To discover whether you have mold toxicity, we recommend consulting Dr. Ritchie Shoemaker's books: *Mold Warriors* and *Surviving Mold: Life in the Era of Dangerous Buildings*. A do-it-yourself preliminary test for mold toxicity, called the Visual Contrast Sensitivity test, can also be found on his website: *SurvivingMold.com*.

Treating mold involves first removing the active fungus with antimicrobial remedies such as pau d'arco, garlic, grapefruit seed extract or various aromatic oils and then eliminating the mycotoxins that it produces with other remedies such as Cholestyramine, galla chinesis and Cholestepure, along with a sugarless diet.

You should avoid all of the following foods while you are eliminating fungal infections from your body. Treatment for these infections can take anywhere from six to eight weeks, or as long as six to eight months, if your immune system is weak.

Foods to Avoid While Doing Anti-Fungal Treatment

- Artificial sweeteners and sugars of all kinds (including honey, maple syrup, agave, xylitol, erythritol, sucralose, aspartame, saccharin, fructose, corn syrup).
- All fruits and fruit juices except lemons, limes, tomatoes and avocados.
- Grains, including the breading on fried foods. This includes pastries, pizza, wheat, couscous, triticale, spelt, kamut, oats, barley, rye, rice, millet, amaranth, quinoa and teff.

- Peas, lentils, soybean products, dried beans, hummus or other legumes.

- Starchy vegetables, including butternut squash, pumpkin, acorn squash, potatoes, yams, yucca, beets, carrots, etc.

- Milk products from cows, sheep, goats, buffalo, etc. This includes yogurt, milk, ice cream, and soft cheeses (hard cheeses made from sheep's and goat's milk are permitted).

- Alcoholic beverages.

- Vinegar products, including commercial mustard, ketchup and most salad dressings.

- Meats with non-meat fillers, such as hot dogs and bologna; most meat loafs and hamburgers from fast food restaurants.

- Pistachios, cashews, peanuts and peanut oil. Also Canola, cottonseed, corn and hydrogenated oils.

- Pork products.

Initially, eliminating these foods from your diet may cause you to feel weak, tired, irritable and brain-fogged (among other things), and to have stronger cravings for the foods that you need to avoid. This is actually a sign that the fungi are dying in your body, so it's important to "ride out" the symptoms until they pass. You may not ever feel completely well on this diet if your metabolic type requires that you eat carbohydrates, but the bad feeling should pass after anywhere from a few days to a couple of weeks.

Following is a list of foods that you can eat while treating the infections:

Healthy Foods to Eat While Doing Anti-Fungal Treatment

- All types of eggs, chicken, turkey and other fowl (dove, pheasant, quail, Cornish game hens, etc.).
- All clean beef products, bison and game-animal meats such as deer, elk, and caribou.
- Small bony fish with scales, especially anchovies and sardines or wild-caught salmon. (Note: Dr. Cowden believes that many fish from the North Pacific Ocean are contaminated with radioactive elements as a result of the 2011 Fukushima disaster in Japan.)
- Non-allergenic hard cheeses made from goat's and sheep's milk.
- All seeds, nuts, seed butters and nut butters, except peanuts, pistachios and cashews.
- All cruciferous vegetables that are steamed for at least five minutes. (Steaming removes any thyroid-aggravating substances.) These include: cabbage, cauliflower, watercress, collard greens, broccoli, Brussels sprouts, kale, and bok choy.
- All lettuces, salad greens, green beans, okra, asparagus, zucchini, yellow squash, summer squash, other non-starchy vegetables; avocados, tomatoes, lemons, limes.
- Lemonade or limeade made from fresh-squeezed lemons or limes and NutraMedix or KAL-brand liquid stevia natural sweetener.

2. CANCER

If you are actively battling cancer, the aforementioned fungal diet is a very good diet for you to follow as well, at least for as long as you are treating the cancer, since cancer feeds on sugars of all kinds—fruit sugar, as well as the glucose that the body makes from grains and other starchy foods. Some people with cancer mistakenly believe that they should only avoid table sugar, but other types of sugar, even the natural sugar that is found in fruit, should be avoided as well.

If you have Syndrome X, doing a pH test or monitoring your weight and paying attention to how you feel after eating are some ways to confirm whether you should include starchy vegetables and grains into your diet.

If you have a type of cancer that is affected by estrogen, such as some breast cancers, as well as uterine and prostate cancer, you may want to also include some cruciferous vegetables in your diet. These include: broccoli, Brussels sprouts, cauliflower, kale, arugula, chard, mustard greens, turnips, cabbage, radishes, collard greens, kohlrabi and rutabagas. These vegetables contain indole-3-carbidol (I3C), a chemical that helps to break down estrogen compounds in the liver, so that there are fewer of these compounds available to stimulate cancer growth.

I have found that most of my patients who have cancer usually do better if they also restrict animal protein in their diets, since some amino acids that are commonly found in animal protein, especially tyrosine and leucine, can stimulate cancer growth. Animal proteins that are rapidly absorbable and digestible, such as soft-boiled or poached eggs, are best for most people with cancer.

That said, I have found that people with lymphomas, sarcomas, myelomas and sometimes melanomas, do better if they include moderate amounts of animal protein in their diets. This may be because such people have a certain metabolic type that requires protein and which is also prone to these types of cancer. —Dr. Lee Cowden

Additionally, it's a good idea to avoid foods that are mucoid (or mucus) producing, such as dairy products, wheat and soy—because these tend to clog up the lymphatic system, and cancer cells more rapidly divide and multiply in the presence of mucus.

Also, when the lymphatic system isn't clogged up with mucus, cancer cells pass more rapidly through the lymphatic fluid, and have a greater possibility of coming into contact with cancer-destroying white blood cells. But if they are trapped in the lymphatic fluid, then it's easier for them to divide and multiply and more difficult for immune cells to access and destroy them.

A low-protein diet is important to follow only while you are actively treating cancer, especially if you have a carcinoma.

If you have adrenal fatigue, hypoglycemia or chronic fatigue in addition to cancer, you may also require some animal protein for your recovery, since animal protein can strengthen the adrenal glands and their production of DHEA, both of which are linked to immune system function.

3. Diabetes and Syndrome X

Syndrome X is a common condition in the industrialized world, especially the US. It is triggered by insulin resistance, which is usually caused by eating the wrong foods, toxin exposure and stress. It leads to high levels of unhealthy fats in the blood, excessive body fat, and high blood pressure. It is a precursor to stroke, diabetes, heart attacks, high cholesterol (the unhealthy kind), arthritis and hypertension. About half of all Americans have some symptoms of Syndrome X or the full-blown syndrome.

If you have cardiovascular disease, you can mitigate your symptoms by taking abundant antioxidant supplements and avoiding oxycholesterol-producing foods.

If you have Syndrome X and/or diabetes, you should follow a diet that is similar to the fungal diet and keep high-glycemic fruits and vegetables and starchy carbohydrates to a minimum. Some people with Syndrome X may be able to include small amounts of starchy vegetables and grains into their diet, if their metabolic type requires these kinds of carbohydrates. Doing a pH test or monitoring your weight and paying attention to how you feel after eating are some ways to confirm whether you should include starchy vegetables and grains in your diet. Test one food at a time, for a period of time, to discern your body's response to it.

4. High Blood Pressure

High blood pressure that is unrelated to Syndrome X is generally the result of one of two things: environmental toxin buildup in the body or stress. If you have high blood pressure, it's important that you remove these toxins and manage any stressful situations in your life, in order to attain remission from this condition.

In the meantime, if you have high blood pressure, it's important to reduce your salt intake—even sea salt, which is healthy for most people. The average no-added salt diet still contains two grams of sodium chloride, because most foods already contain salt in them.

Besides this restriction, people with high blood pressure who don't have Syndrome X can generally eat all of the types of healthy food recommended in the first part of this book.

Most doctors prescribe magnesium chloride and potassium chloride for high blood pressure, but this is a mistake! The mainstream medical community contends that it's the sodium in sodium chloride that causes elevated blood pressure, but it's really the chloride. So magnesium chloride can elevate blood pressure, as can potassium chloride, and make the problem worse. Magnesium and potassium are helpful for lowering high blood pressure, but only if they are the right kinds.

5. Cardiovascular Disease

Hardening of the Arteries

Most people who have had a stroke, been diagnosed with coronary artery disease, or who suffer from claudication (which is cramping in the lower leg caused by blocked arteries in the leg), are usually unaware that their dietary habits play a role in their recovery from these conditions.

If you have cardiovascular disease, you can mitigate your symptoms by taking abundant antioxidant supplements and avoiding oxycholesterol-producing foods. Oxycholesterol is found in scrambled eggs, omelettes, processed foods and the unhealthy oils that we mentioned in the first part of this book. Transfats, which are found in margarine, hydrogenated oils, and processed foods, can also worsen cardiovascular disease and should therefore be avoided.

Hardening of the arteries (atherosclerosis) is the most common type of cardiovascular disease in the US. It results from eating inflammatory and allergenic foods.

Dean Ornish, MD, president and founder of the non-profit Preventive Medicine Research Institute in Sausalito, California, as well as Clinical Professor of Medicine at the University of California, San Francisco, wrote Dr. Dean Ornish's *Program for Reversing Heart Disease: The Only System Scientifically Proven to Reverse Heart Disease Without Drugs or Surgery.* In this book, he describes how to reverse atherosclerotic disease with diet and stress reduction techniques.

Atherosclerosis is a condition in which the interior wall of an artery thickens as a result of an accumulation of fatty materials and clotting materials there, especially oxycholesterol and fibrin. These materials are often collectively referred to as plaque.

Basically, Dr. Ornish discovered that if his patients went on a strict vegetarian diet and meditated daily, they could reduce the plaque in their coronary arteries by about five percent per year. Conversely, he found that if they followed the American

Heart Association's recommended diet, their plaque levels
increased by about five percent per year! This statistic indicates
that the American Heart Association diet is ineffective for
preventing the progression of plaque formation.

Around 1990, I started seeing patients with advanced coronary and carotid disease. Carotid disease refers to a plaque
blockage in the artery that carries blood from the chest
through the neck (beneath the jawbone) and into the brain.

Most of my patients didn't want to undergo surgery, and were
open to the idea of reducing the plaque in their arteries just by
manipulating their diets and supplemental nutrient intake.

So I put them on a program that consisted of a predominantly
vegetarian, oxycholesterol-free diet, proteolytic enzymes
(which they were to take 30 minutes before meals); magnesium, a variety of antioxidants, such as Vitamins C and E;
bioflavonoids and r-lipoic acid; amino acids such as L-lysine
and L-proline, and a few herbs, such as hawthorne berry
and ginkgo biloba—the latter to improve blood flow throughout the body. I also had them do various stress reduction
techniques.

By having my patients combine a healthy diet with supplemental nutrients and relaxation techniques, I was usually able
to get their plaque levels lowered by more than fifty percent
in just four months' time. It isn't necessary for most people
with coronary or carotid artery disease to have to endure
stents, angioplasty and artery surgery.   —Dr. Lee Cowden

Hardening of the arteries (atherosclerosis) is the most common type of cardiovascular disease in the US. It results from eating inflammatory and allergenic foods.

The allopathic, or conventional medical community believes that this condition is caused by elevated cholesterol. But a C-reactive protein test, which measures inflammation, is more accurate than any type of cholesterol or lipid measurement test for predicting whether or not you will have a heart attack.

Nowadays, many people have adrenal fatigue—which is also sometimes referred to as "burnout syndrome."

Statin drugs, which some people take for high blood cholesterol, lower inflammation a bit, but they cause a variety of other undesirable conditions, including cardiomyopathy, which is a severe weakening of the heart muscle.

You can reduce inflammation in your heart and the rest of your body by eating the right foods and taking herbs such as turmeric and boswellia; doing stress reduction techniques, taking heart-supportive nutritional supplements and grounding your body to the earth on a daily basis (for more information on grounding, visit the site: *EarthingInstitute.net*).

These are less harmful and more effective ways to reduce inflammation than taking a statin drug, which can cause crippling musculoskeletal pain, diabetes, heart muscle deterioration, congestive heart failure, arrhythmias and even death.

Stephen Sinatra, MD, a well-respected physician in the integrative medical community, wrote a book called *The Cholesterol Myth*, which is a worthwhile read for anyone who wants to learn the truth about the relationship between heart disease and cholesterol.

Congestive Heart Failure and Cardiomyopathy

If you have congestive heart failure or cardiomyopathy, which is a severe weakening of the heart muscle, you should also avoid excessive salt (sodium chloride) intake and supplement your diet with Coenzyme-Q10, L-carnitine, D-ribose and a healthy, bioavailable form of magnesium such as magnesium citrate or malate. Avoid magnesium chloride. Once your body's levels of these nutrients are restored to normal and your symptoms have improved, then you can add some salt back into your diet.

Besides restricting your salt intake, you should aim to follow a diet that is appropriate for your metabolic type and according to the guidelines outlined in the first part of this book.

6. ADRENAL FATIGUE/HYPOGLYCEMIA

So far, all of the conditions that we have described are worsened by sugars of all kinds, and adrenal fatigue and hypoglycemia are no exception. Nowadays, many people have adrenal fatigue—which is also sometimes referred to as "burnout syndrome."

It is characterized by fatigue, especially in the morning; brain fog, depression, anxiety, sensitivity to minor stressors; orthostatic hypotension (blood pressure that drops upon standing), insomnia, low blood pressure, blood sugar fluctuations and gastrointestinal problems, along with other symptoms, such as musculoskeletal pain.

It results from living in "fight or flight" or "fast-forward" mode, as well as from our toxic food and environment.

If you have adrenal fatigue, it's a good idea to eat small, frequent meals about every three to four hours. Eating infrequently and in large amounts will further stress the adrenal glands.

Emotional and physical trauma, especially in childhood and when prolonged, is another major cause of adrenal fatigue.

Some healthcare practitioners, such as the late Gerald Poesnecker, ND, founder of the Clymer Healing Center in Quakertown, PA, have believed that chronic fatigue syndrome and fibromyalgia—which aren't really illnesses but groupings of symptoms—are caused in large part by adrenal fatigue. For anyone who wishes to learn more about this condition, Dr. Lam's 2012 book, *Adrenal Fatigue Syndrome,* provides comprehensive insights into the diagnosis and treatment of this condition.

If you know that you have adrenal fatigue, hypoglycemia, or low blood sugar (the latter of which is commonly caused by adrenal fatigue), it's essential that you avoid foods that "spike" or quickly raise your blood sugar. This includes most fruits, high-glycemic grains, natural and synthetic sugars, as well as coffee, tea and other stimulants. The worst offenders are brown and white rice, tropical fruits, white potatoes, desserts, pastries and coffee.

If you must have a sugary dessert, always eat it after a meal containing animal protein, to blunt the blood sugar spike that results whenever you eat these foods by themselves. This is very important because frequent blood sugar spikes and the hypoglycemia that follows from such spikes can lead to insulin resistance and over time, diabetes and/or Syndrome X.

People with adrenal fatigue typically do best on a diet that contains generous portions of healthy fatty foods, such as nuts and nut butters, as well as animal protein, and low-glycemic carbohydrates. Non-starchy vegetables and some dairy products from sheep and goats' milk are healthy for most, as is the occasional non-gluten grain and starchy vegetable, when eaten in moderation and generally with fats or animal protein.

Most food that adversely affects the adrenals, will also affect the thyroid, and vice versa.

If you have adrenal fatigue, it's also a good idea to eat small, frequent meals about every 3-4 hours. Eating infrequently and in large amounts will further stress the adrenal glands. Having a protein snack before bed-time is also a good idea, as is starting the day with some heavily salted animal protein, such as turkey bacon.

People with adrenal gland burnout are often, metabolically, "protein types" and can actually become more pH imbalanced if they eat too many of the wrong kind of vegetables or carbo-hydrates. For this reason, it's important to discern your body's responses to different foods and verify these with a pH test (pH testing is described in Chapter Seven, *Food Combining Techniques for Optimal Digestion*).

An under-functioning or diseased liver can also cause or contribute to hypoglycemia. The liver is the body's primary organ for storing glycogen, which is a type of sugar that your body releases whenever your blood sugar gets low. So if your liver is overtaxed, then it won't be able to store as much glycogen as your body needs when your blood sugar gets low, which can cause or worsen hypoglycemia.

If you suspect that you have compromised liver function, detoxifying and strengthening your liver is important. Herbal remedies such as NutraMedix's burbur and parsley, as well as other well-known liver supportive products, such as liposomal L-glutathione and milk-thistle, can help to accomplish this. Doing coffee enemas and juicing beets and dandelion greens is also helpful.

Finally, healthcare practitioners through the ages have observed that anger is often stored in the liver and gallbladder, and that this stored emotion can lead to a malfunctioning liver. So it's a good idea to forgive anyone that you are angry with, as this can literally help your liver to perform better! In the first book in this series, *Create a Toxin-Free Body & Home Starting Today*, we describe a technique for releasing rage from the liver.

7. Hypothyroidism

If you have hypothyroidism, the same wisdom to avoid inflammatory foods applies. Also, you'll want to avoid eating cruciferous vegetables raw. Some common cruciferous vegetables include:

turnips, broccoli, kale, Brussels sprouts and cauliflower. Raw cruciferous vegetables contain substances called goitrogens, which suppress thyroid function.

Fortunately, steaming these vegetables for more than five minutes will neutralize most of the thyroid-suppressive goitrogens. Peanuts, peanut butter and pine nuts also contain goitrogens, which is another reason to avoid these.

> Raw foods seem to require a lot of energy to digest, and chronically ill people often don't have a lot of energy to begin with. Such people might do better eating a combination of raw and cooked foods.

You may also want to avoid high-glycemic foods that can spike your blood sugar. This includes table sugar, breads, pasta, pastries and starchy vegetables, as well as some high-glycemic fruits such as bananas. You should also avoid coffee and other stimulants. These foods exhaust the adrenal glands, which then affects the thyroid because adrenal function is closely linked to thyroid gland function. When one of these glands malfunctions, the other one often does, too.

This means that any food that adversely affects the thyroid or adrenals, will also affect the other gland, and vice versa. For more information on the relationship between thyroid and adrenal function, we recommend reading Janie Bowthorpe's book *Stop the Thyroid Madness*. Therefore, if you have hypothyroidism, it's sometimes beneficial to follow a diet similar to the one that we outlined for adrenal exhaustion, especially if your hypothyroidism is caused primarily, or in part, by adrenal exhaustion.

8. Chronic Lyme Disease

Chronic Lyme disease, which is an epidemic illness in the United States and Canada, with hundreds of thousands of new cases diagnosed yearly, is difficult to treat. Fortunately, the multiple bacterial, viral and parasitic infections involved in chronic Lyme disease are more easily eliminated from the body when anti-microbial treatments are supported by the proper diet.

Lyme microbes (*Borrelia* bacteria and associated co-infections), like cancer and other infections, are fed by sugars of all types. Most people with Lyme disease also have a damaged gastrointestinal tract and cannot digest grains or dairy products without experiencing inflammation.

According to Ann Louise Gittleman, in her book *Guess Who Came to Dinner?* more than 90 percent of the US population has some type of parasitic infection.

Therefore, if you have Lyme disease and are very sick, you may fare best on a diet that is similar to the fungal diet. If you are relatively functional, you may also do well on a diet that includes some low and medium-glycemic (low sugar) fruits, such as grapefruit, lemon, limes, berries, pears and apples; starchy vegetables such as sweet potatoes, acorn and winter squash; and an occasional serving of non-gluten grains and/or legumes such as brown rice, quinoa, spelt, millet, lentils and beans.

If your metabolic type requires some carbohydrates, you may need to include a few fruits, starchy veggies and the occasional grain into your diet, but in general, most people with chronic Lyme disease feel better and heal faster if they emphasize animal protein, green salads, nuts, nut butters and non-starchy vegetables in their diets.

> Throughout my own battle with chronic Lyme disease, I found that I felt my best on a diet that included non-starchy vegetables, nuts, clean animal protein, and about three to four servings per week of non-gluten grains and legumes, especially quinoa, beans, peas, sweet potatoes, squash and brown rice, along with modest amounts of sheep/goat's cheese and yogurt.
>
> Rarely could I tolerate grains more often than that, but completely eliminating them was difficult, since my metabolic type requires some carbohydrates. Yet I also realized that I would have a hard time getting rid of the infections if I consumed a lot of carbohydrates, so I looked for a happy medium of providing my body with a few food items that would help to boost my energy, while also avoiding, as much as possible, foods that I knew would feed the infections.
>
> —Connie Strasheim

Raw vegetables can also be challenging for people with chronic Lyme disease to process, since people with Lyme disease tend to have stomach acid deficiencies. Also, raw foods seem to require a lot of energy to digest, and chronically ill people often don't have a lot of energy to begin with.

On the other hand, soft, squishy foods such as dairy products and grains (especially gluten-containing grains), which may seem easier for the stomach to process, also compromise digestion, especially when eaten with animal protein, and can cause inflammation. Therefore, if you have chronic Lyme disease, you should eat these foods only in moderation, or avoid them entirely.

9. Chronic Fatigue Syndrome/Fibromyalgia

If you have chronic fatigue syndrome, you'll want to follow a diet that is similar to the one outlined for adrenal fatigue, hypoglycemia, fungus, or even Lyme disease, since most people with chronic fatigue syndrome actually have undiagnosed Lyme disease as well as adrenal fatigue.

Symptoms of all of these health conditions overlap with one another and people with chronic fatigue tend to feel at their best on a diet that is rich in healthy fat and animal protein, and low in grains, fruit, dairy products, starchy veggies and legumes. Fresh, raw foods, especially if they are sprouted or fermented, are often quite beneficial.

If you have either fibromyalgia or chronic fatigue, you'll also want to take special care to avoid boxed, canned and processed foods—as well as any foods that have lots of artificial additives and preservatives, as these cause inflammation and worsen symptoms.

If you have fibromyalgia, nightshade vegetables will also worsen inflammation, so you'll want to avoid these, too.

10. Parasitic Infections

According to Ann Louise Gittleman, in her book *Guess Who Came to Dinner?*, more than 90 percent of the US population has some type of parasitic infection. Yet the popular belief is (still) that parasites are a third world phenomenon. Unfortunately, our unhealthy eating and food hygiene habits, food preparation methods, and contaminated water and food supply have made parasitic infections common in the US and other industrialized nations.

Diatomaceous earth is a powerful nutritional supplement comprised of calcified, prehistoric, microscopic algae that are capable of killing off worms, and is a helpful adjunct to any parasite regimen.

Many types of parasites can infect humans. Protozoa comprise the majority of parasites, and are microscopic organisms that are invisible to the naked eye. They can cause great damage as they multiply and invade the body. Amoebas, giardia, blastocystis hominis, babesia, toxoplasma and plasmodium (the microbe that causes malaria) are some examples of protozoa. Among the larger types of parasites are nematodes (such as roundworms, pinworms, filaria, and hookworms) and trematoda, which are flatworms (including flukes and tapeworms).

Parasites enter the body principally through the mouth or skin, and are transmitted through water (tap water as well as water from lakes, ponds, and streams), contaminated or uncooked food, soil, pets, sexual contact, and fecal matter. From their point of entry in the body, parasites migrate and reproduce throughout the body.

Parasites can live just about anywhere. They aren't limited to the gastrointestinal tract. Many live in the brain, pancreas, liver, heart and other organs—even in muscle and connective tissue, so it's difficult to provide a comprehensive list of symptoms of parasitic infection.

Some of the most common symptoms include: constipation, diarrhea, gas and bloating, joint and muscle aches and pains; anemia, allergies, skin conditions, nervousness, sleep disturbances, teeth grinding, fatigue, and immune dysfunction.

Parasites can cause chronic fatigue syndrome, fibromyalgia, hypoglycemia, depression, and other chronic health conditions. Parasites that live in the gastrointestinal tract commonly cause food allergies and irritable bowel syndrome and also contribute to Crohn's disease and colitis.

Removing parasitic infections is essential for wellness. It is beyond the scope of this book to describe parasite diagnosis and treatment, but we recommend consulting Ann Louise Gittleman's book, or Simon Yu's book *Accidental Cure,* for more information.

Many of us crave certain foods when we are trying to get an emotional need met. If you suffer from depression, you may crave unhealthy fatty and sugary foods, as well as carbohydrates such as bread and pasta.

Dr. Omar Amin in Phoenix, Arizona, offers some of the most comprehensive and accurate testing for parasites, as well as an online symptom questionnaire to help you determine whether parasites are causing your current health problems. For more information on these tests, visit: *ParasiteTesting.com.*

Because there are many types of parasites, the type of diet that you should follow during parasite treatment depends on the infection(s) that you have.

For instance, if you have been diagnosed with a type of worm, avoiding animal protein can help you to eliminate worm infections faster since worms subsist on animal protein. If you have been diagnosed with a protozoal parasite, such as an amoeba, giardia, and/or Babesia (the latter is a Lyme disease co-infection), then you'll want to avoid sugar, including the natural sugars that are found in grains and fruits, since protozoa feed on sugar.

Most of us have some worms and protozoa in our bodies, which are causing us to function at a less than optimal level, so it's a good idea to get rid of them!

Ideally, it's best to first remove any worms from your body with some food-grade diatomaceous earth at the same time that you treat the worms with other antimicrobial remedies. Diatomaceous earth is a powerful nutritional supplement comprised of calcified, prehistoric, microscopic algae that are capable of killing off worms, and is a helpful adjunct to any parasite regimen.

Food-grade diatomaceous earth can be purchased at a variety of online nutritional supplement retailers. It is best taken on a rotating schedule of five days on, two days off, for at least three to four weeks while you are concurrently doing other parasite treatments.

After a minimum of three to four weeks of worm treatment, you can reintroduce animal protein back into your diet. If you also have a protozoal infection, you'll then want to avoid sugars, fruits and simple carbohydrates such as grains and starchy vegetables while you treat the protozoa.

Many herbal remedies will effectively remove protozoa, depending on the type of infection that you have. Some popular remedies for protozoa include: black walnut, wormwood and elecampane, but we recommend that you get tested and follow a regimen prescribed by an experienced integrative doctor when removing parasites. Parasite removal is not a do-it-yourself treatment!

Once you have the bugs removed, you can then follow a diet that is ideal for your metabolic type, and which is in alignment with the other guidelines that we present throughout this book.

11. Depression

Many of us crave certain foods when we are trying to get an emotional need met. If you suffer from depression, you may crave unhealthy fatty and sugary foods, as well as carbohydrates such as bread and pasta. This is because these foods have mood-enhancing effects and provide a temporary serotonin boost. Serotonin is a brain chemical that helps to regulate mood.

Unfortunately, eating these foods can, over time, exacerbate the depression, so if you find that you eat for comfort or to get relief from depression, you may want to get an amino acid and/ or a neurotransmitter profile test done by a competent integrative medical doctor or other holistic physician. These tests reveal nutrient deficiencies that cause depression and provide insights into the types of amino acids and other nutrients that your body and mind need to heal, so that you won't continually crave unhealthy foods.

Therapies such as the Emotional Freedom Technique: *EmoFree.com*, Thought Field Therapy: *RogerCallahan.com*, Rubimed Therapy: *Terra-Medica.com*, EVOX: *Zyto.com/EVOX.html* and EMDR: *EMDR.com* can provide insights and healing from emotional issues that lead to unhealthy food cravings.

Most conventional medical doctors don't do these kinds of tests, but many integrative and naturopathic doctors will. They can then recommend amino acid and other nutritional supplements to help make up for what your body isn't producing or receiving through food, based on the results of these tests.

Some common amino acid supplements that help to heal depression and/or anxiety include: L-tryptophan and 5-HTP, which are involved in serotonin production; phenylalanine and L-tyrosine, which are involved in DOPA, dopamine, epinephrine and norepinephrine production; and GABA and glutamine, just to name a few.

The body also needs certain vitamins, minerals and other cofactor nutrients to convert these amino acids into neurotransmitters. Such cofactors include SAMe, Vitamin B-6 (or P5P), zinc, Vitamin C, magnesium, creatine and methyl-folate.

Some foods contain these amino acids, so it's also helpful to include such foods into your diet once you know what your amino acid deficiencies are. For instance, turkey, pumpkin seeds and cottage cheese contain tryptophan, and GABA and glutamine are found in red meats.

Years ago, nutritional supplements weren't necessary for maintaining optimal health, as our food supply provided all of the nutrients that we needed. But not anymore! As we mentioned in Part One, most foods today contain less than half of the nutrients that they did 50 years ago, which means that most of us will need to take supplements in order to remain healthy, even if we eat organic food. Otherwise, over time, we'll find ourselves deficient in nutrients and susceptible to disease. If you already have a health problem or illness, taking supplements could be vital for your recovery.

If you suspect that you are eating unhealthy sugary foods because you're depressed, it can be helpful to ask yourself whether you are truly hungry, or just emotionally hungry. Often we crave certain foods when we lack nurturing in our lives, or because we want to insulate ourselves from pain. In this regard, food cravings can be a helpful signal to us that we need to heal or change something in our lives. Examples of therapies that can help to uncover and heal the root emotional issues behind food cravings include:

Headaches commonly result from food allergies or sensitivities, especially artificial additives and preservatives. MSG is a common offender and cause of headaches in some people.

- The Emotional Freedom Technique: *EmoFree.com*
- Thought Field Therapy: *RogerCallahan.com*

- Rubimed Therapy: *Terra-Medica.com*
- EVOX: *Zyto.com/EVOX.html*
- EMDR: *emdr.com*

If you suffer from depression, it's also a good idea to avoid gluten-containing foods, such as wheat, and any allergenic foods, since such foods exacerbate depression.

12. GOUT

Gout is a type of arthritis that occurs when uric acid builds up in the blood and joints, and causes inflammation in the joints. Gout can be acute or chronic. When it is chronic, a person has repeated episodes of pain and inflammation and multiple joints are usually affected. Even though conventional doctors don't usually realize it, gout is commonly caused by fungal infections, so if you have this condition, you may want to follow the fungal diet outlined in the first part of this book to see if your symptoms improve. You should also avoid organ meats, which are high in uric acid.

13. OXYLATE EXCESS AND INTOLERANCE

Oxylates are a natural chemical that is found in high amounts in some fruits, including berries such as strawberries, currants, blackberries and raspberries; tangerines, kiwis, and concord grapes. They are also found in leafy green veggies such as collard and dandelion greens; beets, potatoes, sweet potatoes, yellow squash, green pepper, okra, spinach, and some nuts, beans and soy products. Bran, fruitcake, cereal, grits, whole wheat bread, coffee and tea also contain high amounts of oxylates.

If you have PMS, avoiding inflammatory and allergenic foods will also help to reduce symptoms. It's also a good idea to favor healthy fruits and vegetables and eat more of these foods and less fatty meat for seven to ten days prior to the start of your monthly cycle.

Oxylates can either be ingested in the diet, produced by the human tissues (possibly as a response to heavy metal toxicity) or by Candida and other fungi growing in the body. Some practitioners have noted that oxylates increase in people who have heavy metal toxicity, especially from aluminum, lead and mercury. The oxylates bind to heavy metals in the body and are not efficiently cleared from it. Instead, they accumulate in the joints, kidneys and other tissues.

A small percentage of the US population can't metabolize oxylates due to a lack of nutrients in the body, enzyme deficiencies and genetic defects. For such people, oxylates will increase inflammation and sometimes cause kidney stones. If you have ever had kidney stones, you may want to get tested to determine whether you have an oxylate excess, and avoid consuming oxylate-containing foods in the meantime.

In addition, it's a good idea to get an evaluation for heavy metal toxicity and fungal overgrowth, and get these toxins removed if necessary to see if your oxylate levels decrease. A urine porphyrin test is useful for this purpose. If heavy metals are present in the body, levels of one or more of the urine porphyrins will usually be elevated.

14. Sinus Infections

Like gout, sinus infections are most often caused by fungal overgrowth in the sinuses and throughout the body. Following the anti-fungal diet, which we described on pages 75–77. Fungal Infections in conjunction with anti-fungal herbal remedies and sinus rinses with aloe vera and saline can often heal the body of this chronic or recurrent infection.

15. Headaches

Headaches commonly result from food allergies or sensitivities, especially artificial additives and preservatives. MSG is a common offender and the cause of headaches in some people. If you suffer from headaches on a regular basis, one way to determine whether your diet is playing a role in those headaches is to avoid all the foods that

Dental amalgams, which are comprised partly of mercury, release metals into the mouth and gastrointestinal (GI) tract whenever we chew and impair proper absorption and assimilation of food.

you suspect to be allergenic from your diet. These are often the foods that you eat most frequently!

At the same time, eat all other non-allergenic foods on a rotating basis, once every four days, while doing the Coca pulse test (which we described earlier, in Chapter Five, page 67) before and after your meals. If your headaches lessen or disappear, chances are, food allergies or sensitivities were the main cause.

16. Premenstrual Syndrome (PMS)

Premenstrual syndrome is principally caused by a hormonal imbalance between estrogen and progesterone in the body. It is usually caused by estrogen dominance, although overuse of progesterone products can also cause symptoms of PMS.

Most women in the United States suffer from some symptoms of PMS due to the abundance of chemical toxins in our environment, which get into the body and cause symptoms of estrogen dominance, since these chemicals mimic estrogen's effects. This excess estrogen-like activity in the body causes symptoms such as fatigue, headaches, depression, insomnia, cramps, bloating, joint and muscle pain, brain fog and weight gain, among others.

You should especially avoid food contaminated by plastic, as plastics have powerful estrogen-like effects upon the body. If you have PMS, avoiding inflammatory and allergenic foods will also help to reduce your symptoms. It's also a good idea to favor healthy fruits and vegetables and eat more of these foods and less fatty meat for seven to ten days prior to the start of your monthly cycle. This will ease your liver's metabolic burden and enable it to more effectively break down estrogen, which in turn will ease symptoms of PMS.

17. Digestive Disorders (Low Stomach Acid, Colitis, and Irritable Bowel and Leaky Gut Syndromes)

Many of us have digestive problems nowadays due again to—you guessed it—our contaminated food supply, polluted environment, chronic stress and lifestyle choices. Pesticides and antibiotics in conventionally produced foods damage the gut and compromise food absorption and assimilation. Antibiotics kill off beneficial bacteria in the gut and pesticides directly damage the cells that line the stomach and small intestine. This in turn impairs hydrochloric acid production, bile salt release and pancreatic enzyme production. We'll discuss why these things matter later in this section.

If you don't have a sufficient amount of hydrochloric acid (HCl), then not only will you not properly digest your food, but your body won't receive the benefit of the nutrients in that food.

Heavy metals in dental amalgams, fish, air and water damage the gut, too. Dental amalgams, which are comprised partly of mercury, release metals into the mouth and gastrointestinal (GI) tract whenever we chew and impair proper absorption and assimilation of food.

Drugs also damage the GI tract. Over-the-counter antacids such as Maalox® and Mylanta®, and acid blockers such as Prilosec®— are examples of commonly prescribed drugs that harm the GI tract and never get to the root of the problem. Instead, they worsen it over time! Prilosec probably harms the GI tract even more than histamine blockers such as Pepsin® and Zantac®.

When you have digestive problems that result from taking these medications, it causes low stomach acid, insufficient levels of pancreatic enzymes, and impaired bile salt release. When you don't have enough of these things, you won't properly digest your food and will even feel hungry after you eat because hydrochloric acid, enzymes and bile salts are essential for food absorption and assimilation.

All of the aforementioned drugs reduce stomach acid production so much that dietary proteins cannot be digested. This causes the undigested proteins to pass through microscopic holes in the intestinal lining and enter the blood stream, where they cause allergies. The allergic reactions then further inflame and damage the lining of the stomach and intestines.

If you have low stomach acid, it's better to supplement your body with bile salts and plant-derived proteolytic enzymes—which help to digest protein—until you can get your stomach lining regenerated.

Also, hydrochloric acid deficiencies cause the gut to become more susceptible to parasitic infection. When there are sufficient amounts of hydrochloric acid in the stomach, this acid will kill parasites that enter the body through our food and drink. Once parasites enter the gut, they burrow tiny holes in the intestinal wall, which then causes leaky gut syndrome, food allergy reactions and allergic gastroenteritis.

If you suspect that you have low hydrochloric acid, you can confirm this with a hair mineral analysis test, which is useful for indirectly assessing stomach acid levels. If your test results show that you are two standard deviations below the normal range for five or more minerals, then chances are your stomach acid levels are too low.

If you don't have a sufficient amount of hydrochloric acid (HCl), then not only will you not properly digest your food, but your body won't receive the benefit of the nutrients in that food.

A simpler way to measure your stomach acid is to do a fasting saliva pH test before a meal, and then measure your pH 20 minutes after the meal. (We describe how to measure your saliva pH levels in Chapter Nine.) If your pH doesn't become more alkaline after you eat, it means that you aren't releasing enough hydrochloric acid into your stomach. Your blood pH and saliva pH should go up significantly immediately following a meal.

Another indication that you aren't producing enough hydrochloric acid (HCl) is if you get full easily or have trouble getting certain foods, such as raw veggies, down at mealtimes. If you eat slowly, or feel heavy and tired after you eat, especially after a small or average-sized meal, these can be other indications of an HCl deficiency. Chronic stress is a common cause of low HCl, so treating this condition will also help your body to more effectively digest food.

When the stomach produces sufficient HCl, it creates a chain reaction throughout the digestive tract. This is because, during the process of digestion, HCl is dumped into the first part of the small intestine. This in turn stimulates the gallbladder to dump bile salts into the small intestine. Bile salts also play a crucial role in food digestion, particularly fat digestion.

So the more HCl you have, the more bile you will release into the small intestine. HCl also stimulates the release of pancreatic enzymes, which also play an important role in food breakdown and assimilation. So the more HCl that you have, the more bile salts and pancreatic enzymes that will be available to break down your food and increase the effectiveness of your digestion.

> For years, I have taught stress reduction techniques to my patients to help them balance their autonomic nervous systems, so that their stomachs would produce the proper amount of HCl, pancreatic enzymes and bile salts, all of which are necessary for digestion. —Dr. Lee Cowden

Most HCl deficiencies are caused by damage to the stomach lining. Therefore, the best way to correct an HCl deficiency is to regenerate your stomach lining so that it will produce sufficient hydrochloric acid on its own. You can do this by taking gut-healing supplements such as aloe vera, slippery elm and/or marshmallow root; removing chemically contaminated and allergenic foods from your diet, and eliminating all infections in your gut with antimicrobial substances.

It's also essential to remove any sources of protracted emotional stress, since stress compromises HCl production. An effective stress reduction technique will be described later in this section.

Some healthcare practitioners advocate increasing HCl pro-duction with supplements, but this is based on a "replacement" mentality, in which the practitioner believes that it's best to simply replace whatever is missing in the body with the equivalent supplement. This is sometimes okay, but in the case of HCl deficiency it's better to find out what the cause of the deficiency is and fix that instead. HCl pills are usually acceptable to take in the short term, but are a bad idea over the long run.

Another problem with HCl supplementation, besides the fact that it doesn't get to the root cause of the HCl deficiency, is that it can irritate the stomach. Many of us who have had the HCl-producing cells in our stomachs destroyed by pesticides, antibiotics, heavy metals and other toxins have also had our mucin-producing cells destroyed by these toxins. Mucin cells are responsible for protecting the stomach lining from hydro-chloric acid, so when you take an HCl supplement, it irritates the stomach lining because there is no mucin to protect it against the supplement.

If you have low stomach acid, it's better to supplement your body with bile salts and plant-derived proteolytic enzymes—which help to digest protein—until you can get your stomach lining regenerated. Most people require enzymes only for fat and protein digestion, but not necessarily carbohydrates, because when we chew we release salivary amylases, which are enzymes that break down carbohydrates for assimilation by the body.

So if your HCl is low you'll also want to take plant-derived digestive enzymes such as bromelain, papain and carnivora, to help your body digest protein, and bile salts to digest fat.

Stress also greatly impacts the effectiveness of digestion. Your body's ability to produce stomach acid is highly dependent upon having a balanced autonomic nervous system (ANS). The autonomic nervous system is responsible for the "automatic" functions of the body, such as breathing, heart rate, blood pressure and digestion.

When you are anxious, hurried or stressed, you throw your ANS out of balance, which then causes all of the body's ANS functions, including digestion, to not work as well.

Also, acid reflux, a condition that occurs when stomach acid backs up into the esophagus or swallowing tube and damages the esophagus, is almost always caused by parasites in the ileocecal valve.

For years, I have taught stress reduction techniques to my patients to help them balance their autonomic nervous system, so that their stomach would produce the proper amount of HCl, pancreatic enzymes and bile salts, all of which are necessary for digestion.

Doing stress reduction techniques can also, over time, stimulate mucin production, which helps to regenerate the stomach lining. Following are instructions for one popular stress reduction technique that I have taught my patients and now teach other doctors to do.

For this technique, you gently hold your left thumb and left index finger together with your right hand. Sit in a comfortable position. Relax. Roll your head around a few times to relax the muscles in your neck. Breathe in deeply and slowly through your nose. Let the air fill your lungs completely. Then breathe out through your mouth, without forcing the air out. Continue doing this for about four minutes.

Then, imagine a peaceful place that you have been to— maybe a vacation spot or a wonderful childhood memory. Remember that place with all of your senses. See the surroundings. Hear the sounds. Feel, smell and taste that place with your mind. For example, if the place that you imagine is a beach, then visualize the ocean, the sand and the seagulls. Hear the waves crashing on the beach and the sounds that the seagulls make. Feel the sand squishing through your toes as you walk, the warm sun touching your body, and the breeze blowing through your hair. Smell the ocean air and taste the salt water on your tongue. Focus on this memory and hold it in your mind for about four minutes.

If you practice this four times a day (before all three meals and at bedtime), you will greatly reduce your emotional stress during the day and will also sleep better and longer at night. Practicing this technique on a regular basis will, over time, allow you to recall it more easily so that you can utilize it at any given time whenever you find yourself in a stressful situation. If you are with others (during a stressful moment), all you need to do is to excuse yourself to the bathroom (if possible) to find a quiet moment alone. Then you can go through the technique, and return to the stressful situation in a better frame of mind.

The stress reduction technique works better if you rub ten drops of Bach Rescue Remedy somewhere on your head, face or neck before starting the first step. Alternatively, you can take 15-30 drops of Nutramedix Amantilla in ¼ - ½ cup of water just before starting the technique.

—Dr. Lee Cowden

So proper nutrition and health aren't just about what we eat, but what we absorb. You can eat a lot of healthy food and not absorb anything.

Many people in the US suffer from acid indigestion symptoms, and buy over-the-counter acid-blocking products such as Maalox, Mylanta and Zantac. These often provide symptom relief but, as previously mentioned, they also destroy the GI tract's ability to digest and absorb proteins and fats. If you take these drugs on a regular basis, over time, the only type of food that you may be able to effectively digest are carbohydrate-containing foods, which can then lead to weight gain, since sugar and starchy foods get converted to fat in the body.

The standard "meat and potatoes" American diet is not a good one for people with HCl deficiencies!

Acid indigestion drugs are one cause of the obesity epidemic in the US. If more people understood that acid indigestion isn't caused by an excess of HCl but rather a mucin deficiency, fewer people would take these drugs.

Also, acid reflux, a condition that occurs when stomach acid backs up into the esophagus or swallowing tube and damages the esophagus, is almost always caused by parasites in the ileocecal valve. The ileocecal valve is a small structure that is found at the junction of the small and large intestines. Treating the body for parasites can therefore sometimes eliminate the need for Maalox or Mylanta.

Some people also take Zantac and other stomach acid blockers to treat ulcers. Most often, however, ulcers are caused by a type of harmful bacteria in the gut called helicobacter pylori. This bacteria thrives in the stomach whenever HCl production has been compromised by chronic stress. If you have an ulcer, we recommend that you get tested and treated for H. pylori (preferably with herbs rather than antibiotics), and follow the suggestions for regenerating your stomach lining, so that your normal HCl production can be restored.

Eliminating any major stress in your life is also important. Doing these things is essential for eliminating ulcers and other GI problems.

CHAPTER SEVEN

About Food Combining and Food Cravings

FOOD COMBINING TECHNIQUES FOR OPTIMAL DIGESTION

Until your digestive processes are normalized and your stomach is producing enough HCl, it's also a good idea to do a few food combining techniques at mealtimes. This will enable your body to make the best use of its limited amounts of hydrochloric acid (HCl) and will maximize the effectiveness of your digestion.

When we combine and eat many different types of food together at mealtimes, the stomach has to produce greater amounts of acid to digest that food. This stresses the digestive organs and if not enough HCl is available, small particles of undigested food won't get broken down and will instead pass through the walls of the small intestine undigested, and cause food allergies and inflammation throughout your body.

To avoid this, it's best to not eat fruit with animal protein or other foods, because that fruit can putrefy in the gut, and impair the digestion of all the foods in the meal.

It's best to eat just one type of fruit at a time, on an empty stomach. You should then wait 45 minutes before eating any other fruits or foods. If you eat fruit after a meal, it's best to eat it several hours after the meal. This is because it takes about an hour and a half for vegetables to be cleared from the stomach; three hours for chicken, other poultry and fish to be cleared, and seven to eight hours for beef to be cleared. So the heavier the meal you eat, the longer you'll want to wait before eating the fruit.

If you have trouble getting raw veggies down, we recommend putting them into a blender or Vitamix, or combining them with fruits into a smoothie. This can help you to get your body's required intake of vegetables.

Also, if you have low levels of HCl (which is a condition that is common among those of us who have been chronically stressed), you'll want to avoid eating starchy foods at the same time as animal protein. This includes starchy vegetables like potatoes, and grains such as bread and pasta. Starchy foods buffer the acids in your stomach and compromise your digestion. The standard "meat and potatoes" American diet is not a good one for people with HCl deficiencies!

Starchy foods also prevent the gut from converting pepsinogen (the digestive enzyme that the body produces for breaking down protein) into pepsin, which the body uses to digest dietary protein. So if you eat meat or other types of animal protein with your meals, avoid also eating grains, legumes, and starchy veggies with those meals. Instead, choose a salad and/or some non-starchy vegetables to eat with your protein.

It's best to eat starches separately, unless you are hypoglycemic or have adrenal fatigue (burnout syndrome), in which case eating a starch by itself isn't a good idea, since it can cause a blood-sugar spike that may make you feel worse than if you had eaten the food with a meat or other protein. If you have hypoglycemia or adrenal fatigue, consider eating starches with a large salad. The non-starchy vegetables will help to slow the rate at which the body converts the starchy ones into sugar.

While everyone can benefit from these food-combining guidelines, they are especially important if you have a serious chronic illness or compromised hydrochloric acid production.

In summary, it's possible to restore your gut and digestion to optimal health, by doing all of the following:

1. Completing stress reduction techniques before every meal
2. Eliminating any parasites and/or other microbes from your gut
3. Following proper food combining principles
4. Taking gut-healing herbs and digestive enzymes
5. Eating a clean, healthy diet

It can take time, but your stomach can regenerate and you'll find that you can eat whatever healthy foods you want, without suffering from ulcers, acid reflux, leaky gut syndrome, and other digestive conditions that afflict many of us today. When that happens, you'll no longer need digestive enzymes, hydrochloric acid, bile salts, or other digestive aids to be well. In the meantime, digestive aids can help your body to absorb the nutrients that it needs to rebuild itself.

What to Do If You Can't Digest Raw Vegetables

Many people, especially those with chronic health conditions involving the gastrointestinal tract, have trouble digesting raw vegetables. Interestingly, everywhere we read, nutrition books admonish us to consume plenty of fresh, raw green vegetables— but who wants to eat raw vegetables two or three times a day, if you can barely get them into your stomach, never mind through your intestines?

Holistic or integrative medical doctors can do vitamin, mineral, hormone and neurotransmitter tests, as well as fatty acid profiles and food allergy tests, to help you determine why you crave certain foods.

By following the gut health restoration tips outlined in the preceding section, you can help your gut to heal so that you can more easily digest raw vegetables. In the meantime, if you have trouble getting raw veggies down, we recommend putting them into a blender or Vitamix, or combining them with fruits into a smoothie. This can help you to get your body's required intake of vegetables. Alternatively, if you ferment vegetables for a few days, this usually improves their digestibility, so eating kimchi may help you to get enough veggies into your diet.

Cooking vegetables in a stew or soup is another way to ensure that you are getting enough vegetables into your diet, and cooked veggies tend to be easier for some people's stomachs to process than raw ones. Cooked vegetables don't have the same nutritional value as raw ones, but if you aren't properly digesting the raw ones anyway, you might as well cook them!

That said, we don't recommend relying exclusively upon a diet of cooked vegetables, since raw ones are more nutrient-rich. But if your digestion is compromised by chronic illness, consider a combined diet of blended and fermented raw and cooked vegetables.

How Food Cravings Can Help You Determine What Your Body Needs

Most of us experience food cravings. At times, these cravings are a signal to our bodies that we need a specific type of nutrient. For instance, if your body is low in tryptophan, which it uses to make serotonin, a mood-enhancing brain chemical, you may crave foods that contain tryptophan, such as turkey or cottage cheese. Or you may crave sugary pastries or bread, since carbohydrates temporarily raise serotonin levels.

Or you may crave sugar when your body really wants a nutrient that is found in fruit—such as Vitamin C or one of the B vitamins.

Or you may crave fatty foods when your body needs essential fatty acids (EFAs). Protein cravings can signal a need for a specific amino acid (amino acids are the building blocks of proteins) such as tyrosine, which is necessary for making thyroid hormone and the neurotransmitters dopamine, epinephrine and norepinephrine.

At other times, food cravings are a sign that your body is actually allergic to the foods that you crave! This happens because when you eat a food to which you are allergic, it causes your body to release a neurotransmitter or brain chemical called histamine which is a pleasure-inducing neurotransmitter. This neurotransmitter triggers cravings.

One principle of metabolic typing is that everyone processes food differently and has a different rate of cellular oxidation, which in simple terms describes the rate at which the body's cells convert food into energy.

If your craving is for a food that you love but which you know is bad for you, you may be allergic to that food. Now, that doesn't mean that your body isn't needing a nutrient that is found in that food, or isn't trying to make up for a deficiency by craving something that provides a similar immediate benefit to what your body really needs, but it's good to determine why you crave certain foods.

Holistic or integrative medical doctors can do vitamin, mineral, hormone and neurotransmitter tests, as well as fatty acid profiles and food allergy tests, to help you determine why you crave certain foods. You can then replenish your body with the nutrients that it needs, and after awhile you will be less likely to crave those unhealthy foods.

So don't beat yourself up if you can't quit coffee or sweets cold turkey! Your body may desperately need a certain type of nutrient that you try to obtain by eating unhealthy foods, and it can be difficult to stop eating those unhealthy foods until that need gets met. We just mention food cravings here so that you know that there is a valid reason why you desire to eat foods that aren't good for you—usually a nutrient deficiency of some sort—as well as solutions for overcoming the cravings.

CHAPTER EIGHT

Eat According to Your Metabolic Type

A BALANCED METABOLISM

Of all the diets that have been developed in recent years, we believe that the Metabolic Typing diet, which was first developed by the Texas dentist William Donald Kelley, DDS, in the 1960s, provides some of the best insights into what we should all be eating.

This diet is based on the premise that every person's body uses water, food and air in a unique manner to maintain life. No two people are exactly the same and everyone has a unique biochemistry, personality, temperament and habits, all of which influence dietary requirements—and that is similar to the premise of *Foods That Fit a Unique You,* as well.

Dr. Kelley believed that tailoring your diet to your body's unique metabolism would push the autonomic nervous system towards equilibrium. This is important as, according to Kelley, the autonomic nervous system has the greatest effect upon metabolism. He defined "metabolism" as the sum total of all the chemical reactions that occur in the body.

> **Through his research, Dr. Kelley identified three main metabolic types that he called vegetarian, carnivore and balanced. They correspond to the three principal types of food on which different people thrive.**

A balanced metabolism improves all functions of the body, including digestion, circulation and immune function, and helps the body to heal from a variety of chronic degenerative diseases. Dr. Kelley linked different syndromes and health conditions to specific metabolic types.

Another principle of metabolic typing is that everyone processes food differently and has a different rate of cellular oxidation, which in simple terms describes the rate at which the body's cells convert food into energy. Cellular oxidation is frequently mentioned as a cornerstone of metabolic typing in other literature on the topic, although cellular oxidation represents just one aspect of Kelley's theory of metabolic typing.

Metabolic Typing

Dr. Kelley developed metabolic typing after he was diagnosed with metastatic (or late-stage) pancreatic cancer. His doctor had told him that he would be dead within 60 days of his diagnosis, no matter what treatment he pursued. Dr. Kelley dismissed his doctor's prognosis and discovered that when he took high doses of pancreatic enzymes orally and made certain dietary changes, his pancreatic cancer reversed. He was fully healed within approximately 60 days of his terminal diagnosis.

As part of his recovery and subsequent work in helping other patients with cancer, Dr. Kelley developed a diet for people with cancer, which later led to the creation of what is now popularly known as the Metabolic Typing diet.

Dr. Kelley's patients knew that he had been given a terminal diagnosis, so when he didn't pass away after 60 days, they sent everyone that they knew who had been diagnosed with cancer to him, and for many years after that, he helped a number of people with supposedly incurable cancers to recover.

In the meantime, he was frequently harassed by the medical establishment, including the Texas medical board, which brought legal action against him for practicing medicine without a license. However, he continued to help people with cancer to recover by having them sign a consent form that stated that he was simply providing them with nutritional advice, and not practicing medicine.

Dr. Kelley's diet for people with active cancer is similar to the diet that we recommend for cancer, in that it is low in animal protein and high in fresh vegetables. But his metabolic typing guidelines are based on a variety of factors, including individual biochemistry.

Three Main Metabolic Types

Through his research, Dr. Kelley identified three main metabolic types, which he called vegetarian, carnivore and balanced, and which correspond to the three principal types of food on which the three metabolically different types of people thrive.

It's a good idea to take Dr. Kelley's metabolic typing diet questionnaire periodically, since your metabolic type can change over time as your body becomes healthier and stronger.

Within these three groups, he identified a number of sub-types (three in the vegetarian category, three in the carnivore category, and four in the balanced category) that are based on individual characteristics. In his booklets *One Answer for Cancer* and *Dr. Kelley's Self-Test for the Different Metabolic Types*, Dr. Kelley defined these metabolic types and the type of diet for each.

According to Dr. Kelley, people who are carnivore types require more animal protein and fat and fewer carbohydrates in their diets than others, while vegetarian types need more carbohydrates than fat and protein. Balanced types require a more even ratio of carbohydrates, proteins and fat. The percentage of each type of macronutrient and the different types and proportions of food that everyone needs depends upon their metabolic type.

In general, people who are carnivore types (also called protein types) might fare best on a diet that contains approximately 40 percent protein, 30 percent fat, and 30 percent carbohydrates.

People who are vegetarian types (also called carbohydrate types) might do best on a diet that is approximately 60 percent carbohydrates, 25 percent protein, and 15 percent fat.

People who are balanced types might need 50 percent carbohydrates, 30 percent protein, and 20 percent fat, although the ratios can vary, depending upon the person. In addition, some metabolic types need more raw foods than others. Since Dr. Kelley developed metabolic typing, other books have been written on the subject, but the guidelines in these books are somewhat different than those of Dr. Kelley's, and may not have the same outcomes and research backing their effectiveness.

Dr. Kelley's booklet *Dr. Kelley's Self Test for the Different Metabolic Types* contains a questionnaire that you can take to determine your metabolic type and the foods that are right for your type. This questionnaire addresses everything from food preferences to how different foods make you feel, to your physical characteristics, behavioral patterns, habits and more. Dr. Kelley's booklets sometimes sell for $100 or more on Amazon, but recently they have been made available for $37.50 on the publisher's website: *TheBookshelf.us/the-books/dr-kelleys-self-test/*.

Since Dr. Kelley is the pioneer of metabolic typing, his self-test may be the most accurate for determining your metabolic type, but if you can't afford this test, Joe Mercola, DO, also has a free Internet questionnaire on metabolic typing which can be found at the following website:

Products.Mercola.com/nutritional-typing/

Dr. Mercola's books *Dr. Mercola's Total Health Program and Cookbook* and *The No-Grain Diet,* also contain helpful insights into metabolic typing, as well as other valuable information about healthy eating.

It's a good idea to take Dr. Kelley's metabolic typing diet questionnaire periodically, since your metabolic type can change over time, as your body becomes healthier and stronger. Whenever this occurs, your food and nutritional requirements will also change.

> Sometimes it's not the foods that you are eating that are wrong for you, but the proportions of those foods. If you eat too many starchy carbohydrates compared to protein or fat in a meal, for example, you can feel worse after that meal, even if the carbohydrate foods that you ate are indicated for your specific metabolic type.

The effectiveness of the metabolic typing diet is evidenced by the testimonials of many who have used it and attained better health as a result of doing it. Nicholas Gonzalez, MD, is a prominent integrative cancer physician in New York who treats late-stage cancer patients using a Kelley-derived food and nutritional program and has seen great success in his patients as a result. Dr. Gonzalez keeps meticulous records on his patients' progress and has also monitored many of Dr. Kelley's patients who have survived ten years or more.

His records and testimonials have demonstrated that at least 80 percent of his patients do well on a food and nutritional protocol that is based on metabolic typing, and most far outlive their initial prognoses. This is amazing, considering that most of his patients have already undergone harsh conventional cancer treatments and have arrived at his clinic with prognoses of just two to three months to live. Dr. Gonzalez' work is another testimonial to the effectiveness of metabolic typing.

In addition, Dr. Cowden used to find that when his patients would eat foods that were wrong for their metabolic type, this would cause an acid-alkaline imbalance in their bodies, and tissue disease. Thus, metabolic typing also correlates with pH balance. When you eat foods that are right for your metabolic type, then your pH should also come into balance.

While metabolic typing can heal the body of some health conditions and help you to feel your best, we believe that it shouldn't be the only factor to consider when you are tailoring a diet to meet your unique needs. In general, we recommend following the guidelines of metabolic typing, after taking into account your current health condition, any food allergies, and your body's saliva pH. Your pH is a good indicator of whether you are eating foods that are right for your type, anyway.

However, foods that are recommended for your specific metabolic type may not be good for you, if you are allergic to them, you become more pH-imbalanced as a result of eating them, or you have a health condition that precludes you from eating some of them. Often, however, the foods that are recommended for your metabolic type are the same foods that will balance your pH and which will help your body to heal from a variety of chronic and degenerative illnesses.

Your personal experience should take precedence over guidelines. For example, let's say that according to the guidelines of metabolic typing, you should be able to eat brown rice, but you feel tired and lethargic after eating it (as would be the case if you have an unrecognized rice allergy or fungal overgrowth in your gut). This means you should avoid brown rice, since how you feel after eating a food is a more important indicator of whether your body needs the food than the food recommendations for your particular metabolic type.

Or, let's say that the converse is true—that your doctor says that you shouldn't eat bread because it's bad for you, but if you eat bread and feel fine, and bread is a permitted food for your metabolic type, then you should eat bread, unless you have a health condition that precludes you from eating grains, such as Lyme disease.

Or, let's say that your doctor recommends a particular food for you that, according to saliva pH testing, causes your body to become excessively acidic, even though it's supposed to have numerous other health benefits. It would be best to avoid that food, because your body is telling you, through its acidic response, that it doesn't want it.

Some questions you may want to ask yourself to determine whether you are eating the right foods include: Am I hungry soon after I finish a meal containing certain foods? Am I generally satisfied after meals? Do I feel tired, energetic, happy or grumpy after I eat this or that food? In the end, how you feel is the best indicator of whether a food or particular combination of foods is good for you.

Sometimes it's not the foods that you are eating that are wrong for you, but the proportions of those foods. If you eat too many starchy carbohydrates compared to protein or fat in a meal, for example, you can feel worse after that meal, even if the carbohydrate foods that you ate are indicated for your specific metabolic type.

Or if you eat too much protein—a steak that is too large, for example—you might also feel poorly afterwards, because your body needed more carbohydrates to balance out that steak, or simply a smaller portion of that steak. Or you might feel poorly because you lack sufficient hydrochloric acid, bile salts or digestive enzymes to digest the steak.

The metabolic diet is very specific and extensive, and it is beyond the scope of this book to describe the different metabolic types and the recommended diet for each here; therefore, we recommend also reading Dr. Kelley's booklets *One Answer for Cancer* as well as *Dr. Kelley's Self-Test for the Different Metabolic Types.*

CHAPTER NINE

Eat Foods That Balance Your pH

ARE YOU ALKALINE OR ACIDIC?

The fasting saliva pH is a measure of how acidic or alkaline our cells and body fluids are. Foods cause the body to either become more acidic or more alkaline. Fruits and vegetables are generally alkalinizing, and most nuts, legumes, grains, dairy products and meat are acidifying. However, these foods affect people differently, depending on their health condition(s), stress level, food allergies and how they metabolize food, as well as their gut flora and genetic predisposition.

> The pH of pure water is close to 7. In order to achieve optimal health, it is essential for our bodies to have a balanced pH that is as close as possible to 7.0 for saliva (or 7.37 for the blood).

Contrary to popular belief, many of us are not acidic, and do not necessarily require an abundance of fruits and vegetables to attain perfect pH balance. For instance, Nicholas Gonzalez, MD, has found that many of his patients are genetically too alkaline, and actually require more acid-producing foods, such as red meat, to lower the alkalinity and balance their tissue pH. Other people, who are predisposed to being acidic, may need more fruits and vegetables to alkalinize their bodies and attain pH balance.

Many chronic, degenerative diseases result from the body being either too acidic or too alkaline, which is another reason why it's important to balance your pH with foods that are appropriate for your biochemistry.

Your body's pH, or its acid/alkaline balance, is the most important factor that you should consider when developing a dietary plan, after taking into account any potential food allergies and your current health condition.

The Importance of a Balanced pH and How Foods Affect pH

If you aren't too stressed in your day-to-day life or mineral depleted, and when you eat foods that are right for your metabolic type and avoid food allergies, your tissue pH is likely to be balanced, but measuring your saliva pH is one way to confirm that you are eating the right foods, according to metabolic typing and other factors. When your body's saliva pH is less than 7, it is said to be acidic; when it is greater than 7, it is alkaline.

The pH of pure water is close to 7. In order to achieve optimal health, it is essential for our bodies to have a balanced pH that is as close as possible to 7.0 for saliva (or 7.37 for the blood).

So if you are, by nature, a meat-lover, and you feel good when you eat meat, then your body is more likely to come into better pH balance when you eat meat. Conversely, if you are acidic and feel poorly when you eat meat, it's because the meat is making you too acidic. In that case, you would fare better on a diet that is higher in fruits and veggies.

Of course, there are some foods that will make most of us imbalanced—such as sugar and cow dairy products. For this reason, we advocate choosing foods that are appropriate for your metabolic type and which don't cause allergies, since such foods are likely to balance your pH. This is a better way to balance the pH than avoiding foods that have been categorized as acidic or loading up on foods that are deemed to be alkaline.

Balancing the pH is crucial for wellness. Many problems occur whenever our pH is imbalanced. For instance, whenever we are too acidic, we cannot properly assimilate nutrients, and our bodies' chemical reactions and electrical responses will be abnormal.

The metabolic enzymes within our cells produce ATP energy for the cell. In order for them to do this efficiently, the body's pH must be close to 7.0, as the enzymes only operate effectively within a narrow pH range. If the cell cannot produce enough ATP energy for its needs, it will die. When enough of our cells die, we also die.

Like Baby Bear's porridge, the cellular pH has to be just right—not too high or too low—since the cell will not survive if the pH is too high or too low. If you have a continually acidic pH, you will lose minerals from your body's tissues, because the body uses minerals to bind to the excess acids in the tissues, and to escort them out of it through the kidneys and bladder.

To find out what your body's baseline pH is, test your pH first thing in the morning, ideally after fasting for 12 hours overnight, and before eating or drinking anything that day. This reading will give you an idea of your overall pH.

Also, your body requires minerals to make its cellular metabolic enzymes function properly, so when your body becomes deficient in minerals as a result of excess acidity, then your enzymes can't work properly. This results in a weakening of the heart and other muscles and blood pressure irregularities. Numerous other biochemical problems are associated with pH imbalance.

Many chronic, degenerative diseases result from the body being either too acidic or too alkaline, which is another reason why it's important to balance your pH with foods that are appropriate for your biochemistry.

Finally, the body's pH, or acid-alkaline balance, is not only affected by the foods we eat, but also by stress and disease. Managing stress and treating any chronic health conditions will help to balance your body's pH, as will eating foods that are appropriate for your metabolic type.

Measuring Saliva pH

You can do a saliva pH test to help you determine or confirm whether you are eating foods that are right for your unique biochemistry.

Before you do this, we recommend that you first follow the food guidelines described in Part One and remove any allergenic or symptom-worsening foods from your diet, and consider doing a metabolic typing self-test to further establish the foods that best fit your biochemistry.

Then, do the pH test to further refine your protocol. If your pH test results suggest that you are imbalanced, then consider testing the foods that you are eating, one at a time, to determine which ones might be causing the pH imbalance.

To measure your saliva pH, simply purchase pH testing strips from an online retailer, your local health food store or local pharmacy. (Few pharmacies carry these strips anymore, but you can still order them from online retailers.) Make sure that the pH paper that you purchase has a measurement range of 5.5 to 8.0 pH, in 0.2 pH increments.

Some types of infection and illnesses can cause the body to be too alkaline, including ammonia-producing bacteria such as Borrelia, which are found in people with chronic Lyme disease.

After you eat a meal, brush and floss your teeth thoroughly, then wait four to eight hours after that meal before testing your saliva pH. You'll also want to avoid drinking any water for at least an hour prior to testing.

To do the test, spit three times into the sink, trash can or toilet. Then spit onto a small strip of the pH paper, taking care to not allow your fingers to touch the part of the paper where you will spit. Wait for about 15 seconds after spitting on the pH paper before reading your results. After about 15 seconds, the pH paper will turn a shade of yellow, green or blue, depending on what your saliva pH is. A color-coded chart that corresponds to a set of numbers on the pH strip container will reveal to you whether your pH is too alkaline, acidic or balanced.

Among the factors that can cause pH imbalances include: acute or chronic emotional stress; eating the wrong foods or in the wrong proportions for your metabolic type; eating foods that cause the red blood cells to clump together; mineral deficiencies and food allergies.

If it is too acidic (this is the most common response), consider which of the foods in the meal that you last ate is most likely to be inappropriate for you. If you don't know, then eat those foods separately, one at a time, to discern your response to each.

Always compare your previous saliva pH measurements with the most recent one. If you notice that over time your pH is getting closer to the ideal reading of 7.0, then it means that you are making reasonable food choices. But if the readings are moving further away from 7.0 and your stress levels have not markedly increased, then you are probably consuming foods that are negatively impacting your pH, so you'll want to find out what those foods are and remove them from your diet. After you do this, you can then re-test your pH to observe the changes.

It's best to measure your pH four to five hours after you eat most types of food, except for beef, bison, lamb and other heavy animal proteins, which take longer to digest. For these foods, it's best to test your pH approximately eight hours following a meal containing these foods.

To find out what your body's baseline pH is, test your pH first thing in the morning, ideally after fasting for 12 hours overnight, and before eating or drinking anything that day. This reading will give you an idea of your overall pH.

The pH test is one way to fine-tune your diet and is a great way to find out whether you are on track with what you are eating. We can provide you with guidelines for how to eat well, but the results you get with pH testing are one way to confirm whether those guidelines are appropriate for you. Ideally, you want your saliva pH reading to be between 6.8 and 7.2. If it is lower, then that means that you are too acidic. If it is above 7.2, then you are too alkaline.

Factors That Cause pH Imbalance

Some types of infection and illnesses can cause the body to be too alkaline, including ammonia-producing bacteria such as Borrelia, which are found in people with chronic Lyme disease. Also, chronically constipated people with bad bacteria in their guts can be excessively alkaline.

If you are chronically ill and pH testing reveals your body to be too alkaline, you may want to get a test for serum ammonia.

Ammonia is a toxin produced by microbes that causes alkalinity in the body. Some toxin binders, such as yucca root powder, remove ammonia and can help to balance the pH, along with antimicrobial treatments, whenever the body is too alkaline.

In the end, your goal should be to balance your pH, whether you are too alkaline or acidic. So if you have chronic Lyme disease, for instance, you'll want to eat healthy foods that will push your body towards a saliva pH of 7.0. Pay attention to how you feel after eating different foods, and whether you have allergy symptoms after eating those foods.

Some diets, such as the South Beach Diet, Paleo Diet and Atkin's Diet—to name a few—may help some people to become healthier, but are inadequate for determining what the majority of us should be eating, simply because they are "one-size-fits-all" diets.

Among the other factors that can cause a pH imbalance include: acute or chronic emotional stress; eating the wrong foods or in the wrong proportions for your metabolic type; eating foods that cause the red blood cells to clump together; mineral deficiencies and food allergies.

Mineral balance also plays a role in pH balance. If you are too acidic, for instance, we highly recommend supplementing whatever diet you are on with trace minerals, which alkalinize the body.

Since diet isn't the only factor that influences pH, we recommend also evaluating any sources of major stress in your life, and finding ways to eliminate those.

CHAPTER TEN

Avoid Foods That Cause Red Blood Cell Clumping

Some foods contain lectins, which are a type of carbohydrate-binding protein that binds to carbohydrate molecules found on the surface of your red blood cells. A single food lectin molecule will often bind to two red blood cells simultaneously and pull them together, which then causes clumping of the red blood cells.

Red blood cells are supposed to travel through the capillaries—the tiny, thin-walled blood vessels that connect the arteries to the veins—single-file. If your red blood cells clump together while in the bloodstream, before they reach the capillaries—then they can't get into the capillary beds and provide oxygen to the cells. The result is inefficient energy production and lactic acid buildup in the tissues, which then causes metabolic disturbances that can lead to cancer, microbial growth, pain and other problems.

> I have found that patients that eat excessive amounts of foods
> that are wrong for their body type tend to have red blood cells
> that clump together, as evidenced by dark field microscopy
> (testing). When cells get stacked on top of each other like
> coins, they can't enter single file into the capillaries like they
> are supposed to, and deliver oxygen to the cells. This then
> causes anaerobic metabolism that leads to acidosis.
>
> —Dr. Lee Cowden

Certain foods tend to cause red blood cell clumping, or agglutination, in some people, especially the chronically ill. Foods and spices that commonly cause moderate to severe agglutination, regardless of blood type or other factors include:

- Allspice
- Beans (of all kinds)
- Cinnamon
- Jackfruit
- Jerusalem artichokes
- Lentils
- Limes
- Mango
- Peas
- Potatoes
- Rye
- Taro
- Tomato extract (but not the actual tomato fruit)
- Watermelon
- Wheat germ and wheat

If you have a serious health condition or chronic illness, we recommend taking an aspergillus-derived enzyme or other type of mixed enzyme that breaks down both carbohydrates and proteins, such as bromelain, 30 minutes before any meal containing these foods, as well as during the meal. This will decrease the chance of lectins in these foods binding your red blood cells together.

Not everyone will experience health problems from red blood cell clumping as a result of eating the above-mentioned foods, but unless you or your doctor has a darkfield microscope to observe what happens to your red blood cells after eating these foods, it's best to take an enzyme whenever you eat them, especially if you have a severe health condition, or feel poorly after eating them.

> Another practice that is catching on around the United States is the development of vacant lot farms. These are small community-owned greenhouses and farms built within the city, on top of buildings and in vacant lots.

A few books have been written which are based on the premise that your blood type is what determines the kinds of foods that will bind your red blood cells together, but scientific research has shown that the same foods agglutinate red blood cells in people of all blood types, with only a few exceptions. For instance, lima beans have been found to cause strong agglutination of the red blood cells in people with blood types A and AB, but not in people with blood types O and B. Therefore, the premise of blood type-based diets is most likely flawed.

Also, we have found that the dietary recommendations in these blood-typing books don't necessarily lead to improvement in well-being, because they don't take into account all aspects of human biochemistry.

What about Other Diets?

Other diets, such as the South Beach Diet, Paleo Diet and Atkin's Diet—to name a few, may help some people to become healthier, but are inadequate for determining what the majority of us should be eating, simply because they are "one-size-fits-all" diets. These diets will work for some people, because they happen to fit their metabolic type or food allergy pattern, but they will not work for everyone. People with certain metabolic types can end up disappointed when they do these types of diets and find their health conditions not improving, because cookie-cutter diets are simply inadequate for many people.

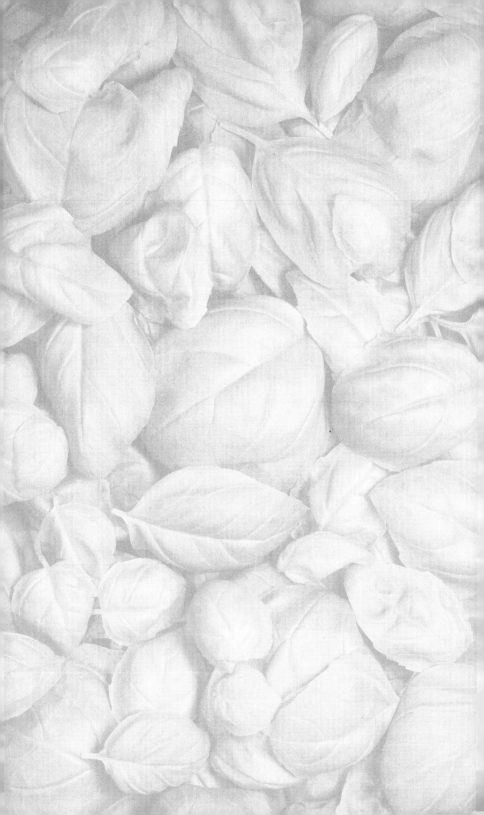

Part Three

*Tips for Food Selection,
Preparation, and
OptimalDigestion*

Nora used to awaken in the morning with her body heavy as bricks. She would down two cups of coffee just to get through the first hours of the morning, but even with the coffee, she battled sluggishness and brain fog—not a good thing for a woman who had to type 70 words a minute, organize meetings and answer dozens of calls daily in her work as an executive secretary. She had also become pudgy in recent years, and often ate on the run. She attributed her mild symptoms to the natural effects of aging and job stress.

She would avoid grabbing lunch at fast food restaurants— because she was aware that eating at these places was an invitation to obesity, since they served meals loaded with unhealthy transfats, but she would still eat out at restaurants.

At night, she prepared frozen dinners made with organic ingredients, which she purchased from the health food store. Still, getting through the day was a chore. Finally fed up with the symptoms, Nora went to a naturopathic doctor, who told her that she might feel better if she changed her diet.

Nora was stunned, thinking that her diet wasn't really that bad. *I avoid bread, fast-food burgers, fries, and sweets, don't I? Why, the organic dinners always include some veggies and healthy meat!*

Her naturopath told her that her adrenals were burned out, and suggested slowly reducing her coffee intake to half a cup daily. She then suggested that she prepare some of her weekly lunches on Sunday night, so that she wouldn't be tempted to eat out at restaurants. While rice and chicken and frozen dinners, in and of themselves, weren't bad foods, Nora wasn't eating fresh organic food. Neither was she eating enough vegetables. The restaurant and frozen food was zapping her energy more than contributing to it.

Nora bought a cookbook and a Crock-Pot and learned how to make fast, but healthy organic soups, salads and stews, using free-range chicken, beef, elk and other meats, along with vegetables and wild rice. She made enough for her week's lunches and learned how to cook simple meals at dinner, using fresh foods.

Nora followed her doctor's suggestions, and within a few months, she had shed some of the extra weight around her mid-section. Her cognition and memory improved, and when she awakened in the morning, she no longer felt as sluggish as before. She attributed these changes, in large part, to her new diet, which included only fresh, organic food, less caffeine, and fewer grains and legumes. By making these dietary changes, Nora's life was dramatically changed.

CHAPTER ELEVEN

Miscellaneous Considerations:
The Benefits of Raw vs. Cooked Foods, Growing Food at Home and Choosing Non-Toxic Cookware

GROWING YOUR OWN FOOD AT HOME

In some towns in the United States and around the world, it's difficult to find health food stores and/or farms that sell organic food. If you don't have access to organic food, or can't afford it, consider growing some herbs, fruits and vegetables at home using organic heirloom seeds.

Even if you live in an apartment or condominium, if you live in a relatively sunny state and have a south-facing window that receives at least six hours of direct sunlight daily, you can grow some fruits and vegetables in buckets or pots inside your home. Just place them in a south-facing window, where they will receive enough sunlight to be able to grow well.

It's possible to construct a 50 x 100 foot greenhouse for only a few thousand dollars. A greenhouse this size will grow enough food to feed up to 40 families.

Make sure to remove anything that would block the sun from entering the room where the food is being grown, such as curtains, blinds or sun-blocking film on or in the window glass. Some trees, such as dwarf lemon, lime, orange and grapefruit trees can even be grown indoors. You can even graft one branch of each kind of citrus fruit onto a single citrus root stock tree.

For more information on how to grow food inside or outside your home, check out the book: *Four Foot Farm: Grow Your Family's Food in a Space Smaller than Your Dining Room Table.* This little book provides a simple design for growing foods in a small space.

The only practice in this book that we don't advocate is growing food in a plastic bottle, since the plastic from the bottle can leech into the food. Mel Bartholomew's *All New Square Foot Gardening: The Revolutionary Way to Grow More in Less Space* is a good book for learning how to grow food outdoors on a small tract of land.

Another practice that is catching on around the United States is the development of vacant lot farms. These are small, community-owned greenhouses and farms built within the city, on top of buildings and in vacant lots. In vacant lot greenhouses, crops are grown in beds above installed water tanks. This practice is referred to as aquaponics farming.

The water tanks, in addition to providing water for the crops, are also used to raise fish. Water from the fish tank is pumped up into the growing beds, and nitrogen, produced from fish feces, fertilizes the plants in the growing beds. Excess water that trickles through the growing bed and which does not get taken up by the plants drips out of the bottom of the growing bed and is recycled back into the fish tank, aerating the fish tank water.

It's possible to construct a 50 x 100 foot greenhouse for only a few thousand dollars. A greenhouse this size will grow enough food to feed up to 40 families. For more information about aquaponics farming, visit: *PortableFarms.com/*.

If you have digestive problems, fermented foods such as kefir, kimchi, raw yogurt and sauerkraut, are excellent choices of food for your gut, because they are already partially digested and contain beneficial bacteria that aid in proper immune function and gut health.

Home-grown food and community vacant lot farms are becoming increasingly popular, as the food supply becomes more contaminated, food prices rise, and people become concerned about food shortages due to political and economic instability. We advocate this practice for all those who are able to do it.

IDENTIFYING HEALTHY FOOD AT THE HEALTH FOOD STORE

While most health food stores offer food that is cleaner, healthier and more nutrient-rich than conventional grocery stores, not all food that these stores sell is 100 percent organic.

I muscle-test foods at Whole Foods, and I sometimes find that some of the foods which are labeled organic, actually have more pesticides in them than foods that aren't labeled organic. This is because the ones that are labeled "organic" have been cultivated on land that formerly was used to grow non-organic food, so there are still pesticides in that soil, which end up in the food.

Conversely, some foods which aren't labeled organic really are organic because they have been grown in virgin soil, but the companies that grow them haven't been in production long enough to be able to complete the rigorous FDA certification process that foods must go through in order to be officially called organic.

The half-life of pesticides in soil is anywhere from 30 to 50 years, so if you want to ensure that you eating organic food, it's a good idea to learn how to muscle test foods when shopping, or get to know your local organic farmers personally, by first name, so that you can learn more about their production methods. Ask your farmers how they grow their food, and visit their farms in person if you can. (Some organic farms even encourage their clients to do this.)   —Dr. Lee Cowden

The Benefits of Raw versus Cooked Food

Vegetables, fruits, and nuts, as well as raw foods of all kinds contain digestive enzymes. Whenever these foods are cooked at temperatures higher than 106°F for longer than five to ten minutes, these enzymes get destroyed, which means that the gastrointestinal tract has to produce more of its own enzymes in order to digest food when it's cooked. Cooking also destroys the B-vitamins and Vitamin C that is naturally found in some foods.

> You can also make enzyme and vitamin-rich soups by steaming a combination of cruciferous vegetables for five minutes, and mixing these with some other raw non-cruciferous vegetables in a low-speed blender until the vegetables become liquid.

One study in which researchers reviewed the findings of about 50 other medical studies on raw and cooked foods concluded that eating raw vegetables reduces the risk of oral, pharyngeal, laryngeal, esophageal and gastric cancers. So it's a good idea to eat foods raw, as often as you can! The exception to this would be meats, since they often contain dangerous, live parasites and other microbes. Cooking kills these microbes, so they are best eaten boiled or baked.

If you have digestive problems, fermented foods such as kefir, kimchi, raw yogurt and sauerkraut, are excellent choices of food for your gut, because they are already partially digested and contain beneficial bacteria that aid in proper immune function and gut health.

Avoid pasteurized dairy products, especially cow dairy, because, as we mentioned previously, pasteurization removes not only friendly bacteria, but also digestive enzymes, some B vitamins and Vitamin C. So, if you choose to eat dairy products, pick foods that haven't been pasteurized.

Today all dairy products in the supermarket are pasteurized, due to US government regulations, but you can purchase kefir starter kits at most health food stores and make your own kefir, or visit a raw dairy farm and purchase yogurt, cheese, milk and other unpasteurized dairy products there.

Although it's best to eat as many raw foods as possible, if you have become accustomed to cooked food throughout your life or have health challenges, you may not fare well on a diet of all-raw plant foods, and may suffer from indigestion, because your gut isn't used to such a diet.

People with sufficient levels of hydrochloric acid in their stomachs can also digest raw food better than those who don't, but putting raw foods into a blender can mitigate this problem. Another advantage to blending raw food is that you don't have to chew your food. Raw food is not as mushy as cooked food, so you have to chew a lot more to break down the plant fibers in raw food, which can be laborious for people

Express gratitude for your food. Studies and experience have shown that this enhances the quality of and body's receptivity to food.

with serious health challenges. No matter your health situation, however, we advocate including some raw plant foods into your diet in order to be as healthy as possible.

You can also make enzyme and vitamin-rich soups by steaming a combination of cruciferous vegetables for five minutes, and mixing these with some other raw non-cruciferous vegetables in a low-speed blender until the vegetables become liquid. Then warm the liquid in a double boiler. If you heat the soup to no higher than 105 degrees (which is slightly warmer than body temperature), it will still contain all of the same enzymes, minerals and vitamins of raw food, because it won't be so hot that it ruins the nutrients, but you'll still be able to enjoy some of the benefits of warm, digestible vegetables.

Healthy Cookware

Just as important as how you cook your food, are the containers that you cook your food in. Until recently, aluminum pots and pans were probably the most popular types of cookware used for baking, sautéing and frying.

When heated, however, microscopic aluminum leeches from pots and pans and gets into the food, and then your body. Aluminum is associated with dementia and other neurodegenerative diseases. The rate of dementia in the US is skyrocketing due largely to aluminum toxicity, which is caused by cooking in aluminum pots and pans, and by using aluminum-containing toothpastes (bauxite), and antiperspirants.

Some people advocate using stainless steel cookware instead of aluminum, but even stainless steel, over time, can release significant amounts of nickel into the food when the cookware is heated. Nickel is also toxic to the body.

Cookware that has a non-stick finish—such as Teflon and Silverstone—releases plastic into the food when cooked, and produces toxic fumes when heated. The results of one study showed that Teflon off-gases toxic particles at 446°F. At 680°F Teflon pans release at least six toxic gases, including two carcinogens. These fumes can sicken people, and cause a condition commonly known as "polymer fume fever."

The best cookware is made from ceramic, porcelain or glass. Pyrex and Corning glass cookware have been known to be more prone to shattering than other types of cookware, so ceramic-coated metal cookware is probably the best type of cookware to use. For more information on healthy cookware, visit: *Cookware.Mercola.com/.*

CHAPTER TWELVE

Optimizing Digestion

BALANCING THE AUTONOMIC NERVOUS SYSTEM

Optimal digestion depends on a balanced autonomic nervous system (ANS). As previously mentioned, the ANS is responsible for the automatic functions of the body such as blood pressure, heart rate, breathing and digestion, which don't require input from the conscious mind.

When our bodies are at rest, in what is called a "parasympathetic" state, then our digestion functions well. If we eat while rushed, or in a "fight-or-flight" mode, which is also called "sympathetic" mode, then our digestion becomes compromised. For this reason, in the following sections, we provide a few lifestyle suggestions to optimize digestion, so that you can get the most out of the foods you are eating, and ensure that the nutrients in those foods actually reach your cells!

Eliminate Distractions

The first way to balance the autonomic nervous system is to eat without distractions. Too many of us nowadays eat on the run. We go through the Drive Thru at a fast food restaurant, or grab a sandwich from home and then eat it while driving.

This isn't a good idea, because when you drive, your body is in a high alert state, and will not properly digest whatever you are eating. Instead, the undigested food will enter into your small intestine and putrefy there. That putrefied food then leaks through the walls of your small intestine, and enters your bloodstream, where it causes inflammation and poisons your liver, then your other organs. Digestion doesn't just affect the gut, but the entire body!

Many nutrients found in food that are essential for health don't get assimilated by the body when it's in a sympathetic state. When the body can't break down proteins from food, it doesn't have the necessary amino acids to make new proteins, which are the building blocks for neurotransmitters (brain chemicals); hormones like insulin, metabolic enzymes, structural proteins to make muscle and skin; and cell membranes (just to name a few).

Your digestion will also be enhanced if you avoid having stressful and distressing conversations at mealtimes.

Cell membranes are sacs that contain the constituents of the cell, and are made up predominantly of fats. If you don't have the right fats in your diet, then you won't get proper cell membrane formation, and your cells won't work properly.

Also, all cells have an electrical charge across their outer membrane that enables them to function properly, but this too gets disrupted when the cells don't have the nutrients that they need to function properly.

As babies, we probably have around -80 millivolts (mv) of electrical energy across all of our cell membranes. By the time we are teenagers, we might have -70 millivolts of energy. By age 40, we might have -50 to -60 mv. By age 70, most of us typically have -40 mv of energy. Whenever we get below -20 mv, our cells become spontaneously cancerous. If we have less than -20 mv of energy in most of the cells in our body, we can die quickly.

A couple of other ways that you can maximize your digestion is by drinking minimal amounts of fluid during your meals (preferably not cold fluids) and chewing each bite of food approximately 30 times.

Yet there are people who, at age 70, have the same cellular electrical energy as a typical teenager because they have maintained a healthy diet throughout their lives. It doesn't matter how old we are chronologically, only physiologically. Proper digestion helps to ensure that our cell membrane potential remains high, so that we don't age faster than we should. It's that important!

Do a Stress Relaxation Technique

Another way to foster a relaxed state while eating is to do a four-minute stress reduction technique before each meal. The technique described earlier in the section on gut problems (Part Two, Chapter Six), is an ideal one for this purpose.

To summarize that technique, simply hold your left index finger and left thumb together in your lap, and grasp your left index finger and thumb with your right hand, while you inhale deeply through your nose and exhale through your mouth. Close your eyes and visualize yourself in a calming, relaxing, soothing place. A former vacation spot is an ideal location. Envision this place with all of your senses for a few minutes— then pray over the food and eat.

Pray and Express Gratitude for Food

Express gratitude for your food. Studies and experience have shown that this enhances the quality of and body's receptivity to food.

I have a US-born Christian friend who lived in the Amazon jungle for eight years and who was invited to eat with the natives several times per month.

The natives had no refrigeration for their food, and would often cook and prepare their meats and other foods several days prior to consuming them. My friend knew that by eating their food, he ran a high risk of getting food poisoning, but he didn't want to offend his native friends, who had shown their appreciation towards him by sharing their food with him. So he would silently pray the following prayer over every meal that he ate with them: "God, thank you for this food. Please cleanse and purify it and prevent it from causing any illness in me or others who consume it." In the eight years that he was with this tribe, he never got food poisoning.

I likewise express my gratitude to God for my meals before I eat and ask God to bless the food because I believe that it helps to provide positive benefit to my body.

—Dr. Lee Cowden

Avoid Distressing Conversation at Mealtimes

Your digestion will also be enhanced if you avoid having stressful and distressing conversations at mealtimes. Don't fight or talk about distressing subjects with your children, either, such as their grades.

How you cook your food determines how much nutrition you will get out of it. We recommend lightly sautéing, baking, boiling and steaming meats and vegetables.

I have found, through my experiences with many of my former patients, that if you talk to a child about something that is distressing to them during the meal, they have a high probability of developing allergies to the foods that they were eating while distressed, and these allergies can end up being life-long.

Seek to have positive, uplifting and peaceful conversations at mealtimes. It will make all the difference in your digestion, not to mention your relationships! —Dr. Lee Cowden

OTHER TIPS FOR ENHANCING DIGESTION

A couple of other ways that you can maximize your digestion is by drinking minimal amounts of fluid during your meals (preferably not cold fluids) and chewing each bite of food approximately 30 times. You want to ensure that your food contains enough saliva for proper digestion, and chewing each bite of food 30 times is one way to do that.

If you drink a lot while you eat, you will dilute your stomach acid and digestive enzymes and they won't function as well. Drinking a lot of cool or cold fluids while eating also causes the gut's blood vessels to constrict so that you can't absorb as many nutrients from your food. If you must have a beverage with your meals, it's better to drink warm water with lemon or warm herbal tea.

EAT FOR HEALTH, NOT FOR TASTE

Many of us are accustomed to eating foods just for their taste. If we don't like the way a food tastes, we don't eat it. But we want to encourage you to eat first and foremost for health reasons, not for the taste of food. Taste is a nice benefit, but tasting food is a momentary thing—which lasts for only as long as the food remains on your tongue. The way a food makes you feel, however, is long lasting.

Would you rather enjoy the taste of a food for five or ten minutes, or enjoy the effects of a food upon your body for a day or more? The Chinese say that we should eat for health first, and if food also tastes good, then it's a nice benefit (but not essential!).

How to Cook Food for Maximum Nutritional Benefit

How you cook your food determines how much nutrition you will get out of it. We recommend lightly sautéing, baking, boiling and steaming meats and vegetables.

Frying and grilling are OK when done in moderation and only if you cook foods in oils that won't oxidize when heated, such as coconut oil. Chemicals that cause cancer and/or hardening of the arteries, strokes and heart attacks are formed when you barbeque and fry foods, so other methods of cooking are preferable to frying and grilling. The less that foods are cooked, the more nutrients they retain.

Never cook anything in the microwave. When microwaved, food becomes toxic to the body. In a study that was done in Germany years ago, researchers put water into a microwave and then gave it to people who had never consumed anything from a microwave before. The researchers then analyzed the subjects' blood and found that bacteria that had been cultured on their red blood cells was fluorescing, indicating that there were radioactive elements in the bacteria from the microwave. The volunteers' blood prior to the experiment did not contain fluoresced bacteria.

Microwaving alters the molecular configuration of foods and beverages, and destroys their nutritional content. There's little point in eating the right stuff if, when you prepare it, you destroy all of the nutrients in it.

The best cookware is made from ceramic, porcelain or glass. Pyrex and Corning glass cookware have been known to be more prone to shattering than other types of cookware, so ceramic-coated metal cookware is probably the best type of cookware to use.

Also, studies have shown that when you cook animal protein in a microwave, its amino acids, from which proteins are made, become altered, and change into a harmful, dysfunctional form that isn't naturally found in food. When these amino acids become incorporated into your body to make body proteins, such as brain chemicals, hormones, metabolic and digestive enzymes, the resultant proteins become defective and malfunction.

Convection ovens will heat food almost as quickly as a microwave, but they are less harmful to the body. Also, microwaves emit harmful radiation when in use and the older the microwave is, the more radiation it emits. This radiation causes cellular damage to our organs if we are in the room where the microwave is operating.

In Summary

By now we hope that you have a better idea about the kinds of foods that will best fit the unique you, and that by following the guidelines outlined in this book, you'll experience increased physical, mental and emotional well-being in your wellness journey. Food is medicine for the body—more so than any medicine or vitamin supplement—so it's important to eat well.

While we have presented a great deal of information in *Foods That Fit a Unique You,* we don't believe that formulating a dietary protocol needs to be complicated. Simply choose clean, natural, unadulterated organic foods that make you feel good and which don't produce or worsen food allergies or symptoms.

Choose foods that balance your pH, and which fit your body's metabolic type. Eat for health, not for taste. Make sure the foods that you eat are real, and in a form that is as close as possible to the way that they are found in nature. Store and prepare them in non-toxic containers made of glass, ceramic, porcelain and (sometimes) stainless steel, and cook them in a way that preserves their nutrients and which doesn't contaminate them with toxic chemicals.

By eating the foods that fit your unique body and needs, you are likely to experience greater vitality, energy, strength, mental clarity, and emotional well-being, among other positive changes. You will probably also find that some of your nagging chronic health conditions will disappear, and that you'll shed unwanted pounds in the process.

Discovering the foods that are best for your body can be somewhat of a trial and error process, but don't give up! Follow the guidelines outlined in this book, and sooner or later, you will get there, and most likely experience better health and well-being than you had ever believed possible.

Further Reading
and References

Academy for Comprehensive Integrative Medicine (ACIM)
AcimConnect.com

"Acid/base balance." *Tuberose.com*. Retrieved on Nov. 5, 2:013 from:
Tuberose.com/Acid_Base_Balance.html

Adams, M. "Microwave ovens destroy the nutritional value of your food."
Organic Consumers Association. Retrieved on Nov. 16, 2013 from:
OrganicConsumers.org/articles/article_6463.cfm

Allen, J. "Canada's oil spill onto the American market." *EMR Labs LLC.*
(2000). Retrieved on Dec. 24, 2013 from: *QuantumBalancing.com/
news/canola.htm*

Almendrala, A. "Prop 37 Defeated: California Voters Reject Mandatory
GMO-Labeling." *Huffington Post*. (2012, Nov. 7) Retrieved on Nov.
18, 2013 from: *HuffingtonPost.com/2012/11/07/prop-37-defeated-
californ_n_2088402.html*

Annual Report of the Pesticide Residues Committee 2008. *Chemicals
Regulation Directorate* (Feb. 10, 2009) Retrieved on Nov. 15,
2013 from: P*esticides.gov.uk/Resources/CRD/Migrated-Resources/
Documents/P/PRC_Annual_Report_2008.pdf*

Barceloux, D. "Potatoes, tomatoes and solanine toxicity." *Disease-a-
Month*. 55, no. 6 (2009 June): pp. 391-402

Bartholomew, M. (2013, Feb. 15) *All New Square Foot Gardening, Second Edition: The Revolutionary Way to Grow More in Less Space.* Minneapolis, MN: Cool Springs Press; Second Edition

Bowthorpe, J. (2011) *Stop The Thyroid Madness.* Fredericksburg, TX: Laughing Grape Publishing, LLC.

Cascio G, Schiera G, Di Liegro I. "Dietary fatty acids in metabolic syndrome, diabetes and cardiovascular diseases." *Curr Diabetes Rev.* (2012 Jan):8(1):2-17.

Casey, J. "The Hidden Ingredient That Can Sabotage Your Diet." *WebMD.* Retrieved on Nov. 15, 2013 from: *MedicineNet.com/script/main/art. asp?articlekey=56589.*

"Comparative study of food prepared conventionally and in the microwave oven." *Raum & Zelt,* (1992): 3(2): 43

Cortés-Giraldo I, Girón-Calle J, Alaiz M, Vioque J, Megías C. "Hemagglutinating activity of polyphenols extracts from six grain legumes." *Food Chem Toxicol.* (2012 Jun):50(6):1951-4. doi: 10.1016/j. fct.2012.03.071. Epub 2012 Apr 1.

Cummins, J. (2001 March) Toxicology Symposium, University of Guelph. Ontario, Canada. Retrieved on Dec. 10, 2011 from: *Psrast.org/ jcfateofgen.htm*

Daley CA, Abbott A, Doyle PS, Nader GA, Larson S. "A review of fatty acid profiles and antioxidant content in grass-fed and grain-fed beef." *Nutr J.* (2010 Mar) doi: 10.1186/1475-2891-9-10. Retrieved on Nov. 15, 2013 from: *ncbi.nlm.nih.gov/pubmed/20219103*

David, D., et al. "Changes in USDA food composition data for 43 garden crops, 1950 to 1999." *Journal of the American College of Nutrition.* (2004) Vol. 23, No. 6 669

De Coster S, van Larebeke N. "Endocrine-disrupting chemicals: associated disorders and mechanisms of action." *J Environ Public Health.* (2012):713696. Epub 2012 Sep 6.

De Lorgeril M, Salen P. "New insights into the health effects of dietary saturated and omega-6 and omega-3 polyunsaturated fatty acids." *BMC Med.* (2012 May 21):10:50. doi: 10.1186/1741-7015-10-50.

De Lorgeril M. "Essential polyunsaturated fatty acids, inflammation, atherosclerosis and cardiovascular diseases." *Subcell Biochem.* (2007):42:283-97.

Divi RL, Chang HC, Doerge DR. "Anti-thyroid isoflavones from soybean: isolation, characterization, and mechanisms of action." *Biochem Pharmacol.* (1997 Nov 15): 54(10):1087-96

Doerge DR, Sheehan DM. "Goitrogenic and estrogenic activity of soy isoflavones." *Environ Health Perspect.* (2002 Jun):110 Suppl 3:349-53

Earthing Institute (for grounding products): *EarthingInstitute.net*

Emotional Freedom Technique: *EmoFree.com*

EVOX: *www.zyto.com/EVOX.html*

Flavin, D. "Metabolic danger of high fructose corn syrup." *Life Extension Magazine.* (2008 Dec). Retrieved on Nov. 10, 2013 from: *lef.org/ magazine/mag2008/dec2008_Metabolic-Dangers-of-High-Fructose-Corn-Syrup_02.htm*

Food Commission, UK. "United Kingdom: Meat and dairy: Where have all the minerals gone?" *Food Magazine.* (Jan.-March 2006).

Ford ES, Giles WH, Dietz WH ."Prevalence of metabolic syndrome among US adults: findings from the third National Health and Nutrition Examination Survey." *JAMA* (2002): 287 (3): 356–359. doi:10.1001/jama.287.3.356. PMID 11790215.

Gittleman, A. (2001) *Guess What Came to Dinner? Parasites and Your Health.* New York, NY: Penguin Group, Inc.

Gonzalez, N. "The Pancreas and Pancreatic Cancer." *Total Health.* (2007 Jan-Feb.) Retrieved on Nov. 2, 2013 from: *Dr-Gonzalez.com/ totalhealth_11_06.htm#diets*

Green, M. et al, "Public health implications of the microbial pesticide Bacillus thuringiensis: An epidemiological study, Oregon, 1985–86." *Amer. J. Public Health* 80, no. 7(1990): 848–852.

Johnson RJ, Segal MS, Sautin Y, et al. "Potential role of sugar (fructose) in the epidemic of hypertension, obesity and the metabolic syndrome, diabetes, kidney disease, and cardiovascular disease." *Am J Clin Nutr.* (2007 Oct);86(4):899-906.

Kelley, William D. (1967, 1977, 1984, 2013). *Dr. Kelley's Self-Test for the Different Metabolic Types.* Litchfield Park, AZ: Kettle Moraine Publishing.

Kelley, William D. (1997 May) *Dr. Kelley's One Answer to Cancer.* Cancer Coalition; 2 edition

Kim JH, Park HY, Bae S, Lim YH, Hong YC. "Diethylhexyl phthalates is associated with insulin resistance via oxidative stress in the elderly: a panel study." *PLoS One.* (2013 Aug 19):8(8):e71392. doi: 10.1371/ journal.pone.0071392

Lam, M and D. (2012) *Adrenal Fatigue Syndrome - Reclaim Your Energy and Vitality with Clinically Proven Natural Programs.* Loma Linda, CA: Adrenal Institute Press.

"Lectins in edible foods & ABO" *Reactions Owen Foundation Website.* Retrieved on Dec. 13, 2013 from: *http://www.owenfoundation.com/ Health_Science/Lectins_in_Foods.html*

Link, L. and Potter, H. "Raw versus cooked vegetables and cancer risk." *Cancer Epidemiology, Biomarkers and Prevention.* (2004 Sept): 13; 1422).

Ludwig, D. "Technology, Diet, and the Burden of Chronic Disease." *JAMA.* (2011); 305(13):1352-1353. doi:10.1001/jama.2011.380.

Make Your Own Yogurt: *MakeYourOwnYogurt.com.*

Maloney, J. *The Four Foot Farm.* Available at: *FourFootFarm.com/ wp-content/uploads/2013/01/1-blue-sky-and-vegetables-different.jpg*

Membrane Potenial. Wikipedia. Retrieved on Dec. 24, 2013 from: *en.Wikipedia.org/wiki/Membrane_potential*

Mercola, J. "Nutritional Typing." *Mercola.com:* Retrieved on Nov. 20, 2013 from: *NutritionalTyping.Mercola.com/Login.aspx.*

Mercola, J. "Why Are Toxin Proteins Genetically Engineered Into Your Food?" *Mercola.com.* (2011 Sept) Retrieved on Jan. 3, 2011 from: *Articles.Mercola.com/sites/articles/archive/2011/09/26/why-are-toxin-proteins--genetically-engineered-into-your-food.aspx.*

Mercola, J. "Genetically-Engineered Soybeans May Cause Allergies." Mercola.com. (2010 July). Retrieved on Dec. 13, 2011 from: *Articles. Mercola.com/sites/articles/archive/2010/07/08/genetically-engineered-soybeans-may-cause-allergies.aspx*

Monnet-Tschudi F, Zurich MG, Boschat C, Corbaz A, Honegger P. "Involvement of environmental mercury and lead in the etiology of neurodegenerative diseases." *Rev Environ Health.* (2006 Apr-Jun): 21(2):105-17.

Multipure water filters: *Multipure.com/mpscience*

National Candida Center website/saliva testing: *NationalCandidaCenter. com/candida-self-exams/*

"News Release: GMOs Linked to Exploding Gluten Sensitivity Epidemic." *Green Med Info.* (2013 25 Nov). Retrieved on Dec. 13, 2013 from: *GreenMedInfo.com/blog/news-release-gmos-linked-exploding-gluten-sensitivity-epidemic-free-pdf1*

Nicholas Gonzalez website: *http://www.dr-gonzalez.com/index.htm*

NRDC Mercury Calculator. *Natural Resources Defense Council.* Retrieved on Dec. 13, 2013 from: *nrdc.org/health/effects/mercury/ calculator/start.asp*

NutraMedix: *NutraMedix.com*

"Open Letter from World Scientists to All Governments Concerning GMOs." (2000) Retrieved from *The Institute of Science and Society: Isis.org.uk/list.php.*

Ornish, D. (1995 Dec) Dr. *Dean Ornish's Program for Reversing Heart Disease: The Only System Scientifically Proven to Reverse Heart Disease Without Drugs or Surgery.* Raleigh, NC: Ivy Books.

"Over 300 pollutants in US tap water." *National Drinking Water Database Environmental Working Group.* (2009 Dec). Retrieved on Nov. 20, 2013 from: *http://www.ewg.org/tap-water/*

Pamphlett, R. "Uptake of environmental toxicants by the locus ceruleus: A potential trigger for neurodegenerative, demyelinating and psychiatric disorders." *Med Hypotheses.* (2013 Nov 21): pii: S0306-9877(13)00543-4. doi: 10.1016/j.mehy.2013.11.016.

Parasitology Center, Inc. (for parasite testing): *ParasiteTesting.com*

Pastori D, Carnevale R, Pignatelli P. "Is there a clinical role for oxidative stress biomarkers in atherosclerotic diseases?" *Intern Emerg Med.* (2013 Sept 22).

"Pesticide-Induced Diseases: Cancer." *Beyond Pesticides.* Retrieved on Dec. 13, 2013 from: *BeyondPesticides.org/health/cancer.php*

Poesnecker, G. (1993) *Chronic Fatigue Unmasked.* Richlandtown, PA: Humanitarian Publishing Company.

Pollan, M. (2009) *Food Rules.* New York, NY: Penguin Group.

Pollan, M. (2006) *The Omnivore's Dilemma.* New York, NY: Penguin Group.

Pollan, M. "Power Steer." *The New York Times.* (2002 March). Retrieved on November 20, 2011 from: *NYTimes.com/2002/03/31/magazine/power-ste.*

Ponnampalam EN, Mann NJ, Sinclair AJ. "Effect of feeding systems on omega-3 fatty acids, conjugated linoleic acid and trans fatty acids in Australian beef cuts: potential impact on human health." *Asia Pac J Clin Nutr.* (2006):15(1):21-9.

"Principles of healthy diets." *The Weston A. Price Foundation.* (2000 Jan). Retrieved on Dec. 13, 2013 from: *http://www.westonaprice.org/basics/principles-of-healthy-diets*

Rice, L. et. al, "Soy isoflavones exert differential effects on androgen responsive genes in LNCaP human prostate cancer cells." *Journal of Nutrition* (2007). Retrieved Jan., 20122, from: JN.Nutrition.org/content/137/4/964.full

Riding, A. "Trial in Spain on toxic cooking oil ends in uproar." *The New York Times*. (1989 May 21) Retrieved on Dec. 24, 2013 from: *NYTimes.com/1989/05/21/world/trial-in-spain-on-toxic-cooking-oil-ends-in-uproar.html*

Rochefort, H. "Bisphenol A and hormone-dependent cancers: potential risk and mechanism." *Med Sci* (Paris). (2013 May) 29(5):539-44. doi: 10.1051/medsci/2013295019. Epub 2013 May 28.

"Role of the insulin-like growth factor family in cancer development and progression." *Journal of the National Cancer Institute*. (2000). Vol. 92, issue 18. Pp. 1472-1489. Retrieved on November 20, 2011 from: *http://jnci.oxfordjournals.org/content/92/18/1472.fuller.html?pagewanted=all&src=pm*

Rubimed Therapy: *Terra-Medica.com*

Sanders D, Kamoun S, Williams B, Festing M. "Long term toxicity of a Roundup herbicide and a Roundup-tolerant genetically modified maize." *Food Chem. Toxicol.* (2012 Mar): 53:450-3. doi: 10.1016/j.fct.2012.10.049. Epub 2012 Nov 6.

Schaller, J. (2006) *Mold Illness and Mold Remediation Made Simple (Discount Black & White Edition): Removing Mold Toxins from Bodies and Sick Buildings*. Tampa, FL: Hope Academic Press.

Sharon A, Sathyananda N, Shubharani R, Sharuraj M. "Agglutination of human erythrocytes in Food and Medicinal Plants." *Database of Medicinal Plants, Karnataka State Council for Science and Technology* (2000 May).

Shoemaker, R. (2011) *Surviving Mold: Life in the Era of Dangerous Buildings*. Otter Bay Books

Shoemaker, R. (2005) *Mold Warriors*. Baltimore, MD: Gateway Press, Inc.

Sinatra, S. (2012 Nov) *The Cholesterol Myth*. Vancouver, Canada: Fair Winds Press.

Strasheim, Connie (2012 Oct) *Beyond Lyme Disease*. S. Lake Tahoe, CA: BioMedPublishing Group.

"Tap water in 42 states contaminated by chemicals." *About.com*. Retrieved on Nov. 20, 2013 from: *http://environment.about.com/od/waterpollution/a/tap_water_probe.htm*.

"Teflon Toxicosis: EWG finds heated Teflon pans can turn toxic faster than DuPont claims." *Environmental Working Group*.(2003 May 15). Retrieved on Nov. 15, 2013 from: *EWG.org/research/canaries-kitchen*.

"The Oxalate Content of Food." *The Oxalosis and Hyperoxyaluria Foundation.* Retrieved on Nov. 3, 2013 from: *http://www.ohf.org/docs/ Oxalate2008.pdf*

Thought Field Therapy: *RogerCallahan.com*

"United States: Vegetables Without Vitamins." *Life Extension Magazine.* (2001, March) Retrieved on March 1, 2012 from: *LEF.org/magazine/ mag2001/mar2001_report_vegetables.html*

Vecchio, L. et al, "Ultrastructural Analysis of Testes from Mice Fed on Genetically Modified Soybean." *European Journal of Histochemistry* 48, no. 4 (Oct–Dec 2004) 449–454.

Wagner M, Oehlmann J. "Endocrine disruptors in bottled mineral water: total estrogenic burden and migration from plastic bottles." *Environ Sci Pollut Res Int.* (2009 May):16(3):278-86. doi: 10.1007/s11356-009-0107-7. Epub 2009 Mar 10.

Watson CS, Hu G, Paulucci-Holthauzen AA. "Rapid actions of xenoestrogens disrupt normal estrogenic signaling." *Steroids.* (2013 Nov 20). pii: S0039-128X(13)00259-6. doi: 10.1016/j.steroids.2013.11.006.

Wolke, Robert L. "Canola Baloney." *The Washington Post* (2001 February).

Wunderlich SM, Feldman C, Kane S, Hazhin T. "Nutritional quality of organic, conventional, and seasonally grown broccoli using vitamin C as a marker." *Int J Food Sci Nutr.* (2008 Feb):59(1):34-45.

Yu, Simon. (2010) *Accidental Cure: Extraordinary Medicine for Extraordinary Patients.* St. Louis, MO: Prevention and Healing, Inc.

Nicholas J. Gonzalez, MD

The author of the Foreword, Nicholas J. Gonzalez, MD, graduated from Brown University, Phi Beta Kappa magna cum laude, with a degree in English Literature. He subsequently worked as a journalist, first at Time Inc., before pursuing premedical studies at Columbia.

He then received his medical degree from Cornell University Medical College in 1983. During a postgraduate immunology fellowship under Dr. Robert A. Good, considered the father of modern immunology, he completed a research study evaluating an aggressive nutritional therapy in the treatment of advanced cancer.

Since 1987, Dr. Gonzalez has been in private practice in New York City, treating patients diagnosed with cancer and other serious degenerative illnesses. His nutritional research has received substantial financial support from Procter & Gamble and Nestle. Results from a pilot study published in 1999 described the most positive data in the medical literature for pancreatic cancer.

W. Lee Cowden, MD, MD(H)

W. Lee Cowden, MD, MD(H) is a U.S. board-certified cardiologist and internist internationally renowned and recognized for his knowledge and skill in practicing and teaching integrative medicine.

He is Chairman of the scientific advisory board and Academy Professor for the Academy of Comprehensive Integrative Medicine (ACIM). ACIM is dedicated to shifting the healthcare paradigm toward wellness by training and supporting practitioners in a variety of holistic health disciplines, conducting research, and implementing therapeutic innovations to create a new global wellness care community.

Dr. Cowden has pioneered successful treatments for a myriad of diseases, including chronic fatigue syndrome, cancer, autism, fibromyalgia, heart disease, Lyme disease, and others. In addition to treating thousands of patients, Dr. Cowden travels and teaches integrative medicine nationally and internationally in countries such as Mexico, Brazil, Peru, Guatemala, Germany, the Czech Republic, Japan, China, Taiwan, England, the Netherlands, Austria, Australia, Norway, Curaçao, the Dominican Republic, Singapore and Malaysia. He is also a member of the Lyme and Autism Foundation scientific advisory board.

Dr. Cowden is the author or co-author of many publications, including the following books:

- *Insights into Lyme Disease Treatment* (2009);
- *Longevity, An Alternative Medicine Definitive Guide* (2001);
- *Cancer Diagnosis: What to Do Next* (2000)
- *An Alternative Medicine Definitive Guide to Cancer* (1997).

Although Dr. Cowden was initially trained in allopathic medicine, early on in his career, he realized that this type of medicine often not only didn't heal his patients but also frequently failed to bring them to a place of wellness and ultimate wholeness so that their illnesses wouldn't recur. With this realization, he undertook a program to expand his knowledge, experience and medical practice to include natural, non-toxic, holistic solutions for wellness.

More than a holistic physician, Dr. Cowden is also a sensitive educator who teaches lifestyle, emotional and spiritual strategies for living well so that his patients can go beyond wellness to wholeness—in body, mind and spirit.

More information about Dr. Cowden and his work can be found on the Academy of Comprehensive Integrative Medicine website: *ACIMConnect.com.*

Connie Strasheim

Connie Strasheim is a medical researcher and writer who has experienced the hardships of chronic illness firsthand through her near decade-long battle with Lyme disease and chronic fatigue syndrome.

Besides coauthoring the books in this series, she is the author of five books on holistic and integrative treatments for disease. They include:

- The best-selling *Insights into Lyme Disease Treatment: Thirteen Lyme-Literate Health Care Practitioners Share Their Healing Strategies* (2009);

- *Beyond Lyme Disease: Healing The Underlying Causes of Chronic Illness in People with Borreliosis and Co-Infections* (2012);

- *Defeat Cancer: 15 Doctors of Integrative and Naturopathic Medicine Tell You How* (2010);

- *Healing Chronic Illness: By His Spirit, Through His Resources* (2010)

- *The Lyme Disease Survival Guide: Physical, Lifestyle and Emotional Strategies for Healing* (2008).

Through her battle with severe chronic illness, Connie learned that attaining wellness isn't just about eliminating infections, detoxifying the body or balancing the hormones—it's about addressing all the factors that caused the body to break down in the first place. These include all environmental, psycho-emotional, lifestyle and spiritual issues that cause or contribute to damage, discontent and—ultimately—"dis-ease" in the body, mind and spirit.

She has also learned, through her experience and research, that in order to be well—never mind being whole—in today's world fraught with stress and toxicity, many tools are required. In this book series, *The Journey to Wellness,* she and Dr. Cowden share some of these tools.

More information about Connie's work can be found on her website: *ConnieStrasheim.com.*

ACIM Press

Did you know that toxins are a primary cause of most chronic and degenerative diseases today, such as chronic fatigue syndrome, Alzheimers, fibromyalgia, heart disease, Parkinson's, irritable bowel syndrome, and cancer? Fortunately, you can heal from your current health condition or simply optimize your health by removing these toxins from your home and body. In *Create a Toxin-Free Body and Home...Starting Today,* W. Lee Cowden, MD and Connie Strasheim tell you how!

First, the authors describe how to identify hidden, dangerous environmental toxins that are found in most homes, as well as in the air, food and water supply. They then describe ways to remove these toxins from the body, using everything from do-it-yourself, easy hands-on manual therapies, to doctor-assisted chelation, oral supplements, and more.

Finally, they teach you how to make healthy lifestyle choices to avoid re-exposure to toxins and to maintain your health and well-being. For more information, visit: *ACIMConnect.com.*

ACIM
The Journey to Wellness Book Series

Create a Toxin-Free Body & Home
Starting Today

W. Lee Cowden, MD, MD(H)
Connie Strasheim

Most diet books today focus on a one-size-fits-all approach to food selection. In *Foods that Fit a Unique You,* authors W. Lee Cowden, MD and Connie Strasheim prove that no two people have the same biochemistry and needs, and that one-size-fit-all food plans are therefore inadequate for determining what you need to eat for optimal health, fitness and weight maintenance.

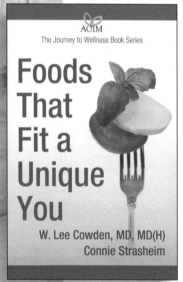

In *Foods that Fit a Unique You,* the authors teach you how to identify truly healthy foods, and look and feel your best, by taking into account six individual factors, including:

- Your body's pH
- Your food allergies
- Your metabolic type
- Your gastrointestinal function
- Foods that clump your red blood cells together
- Your current health condition

In *Foods that Fit a Unique You,* the authors provide general guidelines on how to identify and choose healthy foods, and then teach you how to find the foods that will best fit your unique body, based on the above factors.

They then show you how to avoid food allergens, optimize your digestion and heal your gastrointestinal tract, so that you can get the most out of your meals. For more information, visit: *ACIMConnect.com.*

Conventional medicine has limited tools for identifying and treating the cause of common, but frequently elusive symptoms, such as fatigue, pain, insomnia, depression and anxiety. Vitamins, herbs and drugs, as well as conventional healing tools, such as surgery, counseling, chiropractic care and physical therapy, often fail to help people to heal from these conditions.

Fortunately, bioenergetic medicine can provide gentle, safe and effective healing solutions when other methods fail. In *BioEnergetic Wellness Tools: How to Heal from Fatigue, Pain, Insomnia, Depression, and Anxiety*, authors W. Lee Cowden, MD and Connie Strasheim explain the advantages of bioenergetic medicine over other types of healing modalities.

They then share the bioenergetic tools that they have found to be most effective for healing the body from five often difficult-to-treat conditions, including fatigue, pain, insomnia, depression and anxiety. These tools range from inexpensive and gentle homeopathic and energetically-imprinted remedies, to powerful energetic devices, do-it-yourself hands-on healing techniques, and diagnostic devices that help to detect imbalances and problems in the body.

Discover the tools that can help you to recover from conditions that conventional medicine has failed to treat! For more information, visit: *ACIMConnect.com*.

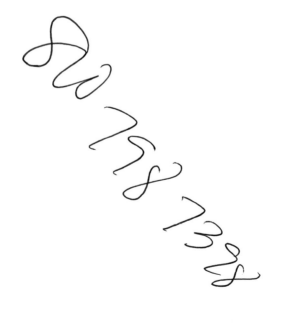